The Essential

DIET FOR DIVERTICULITIS

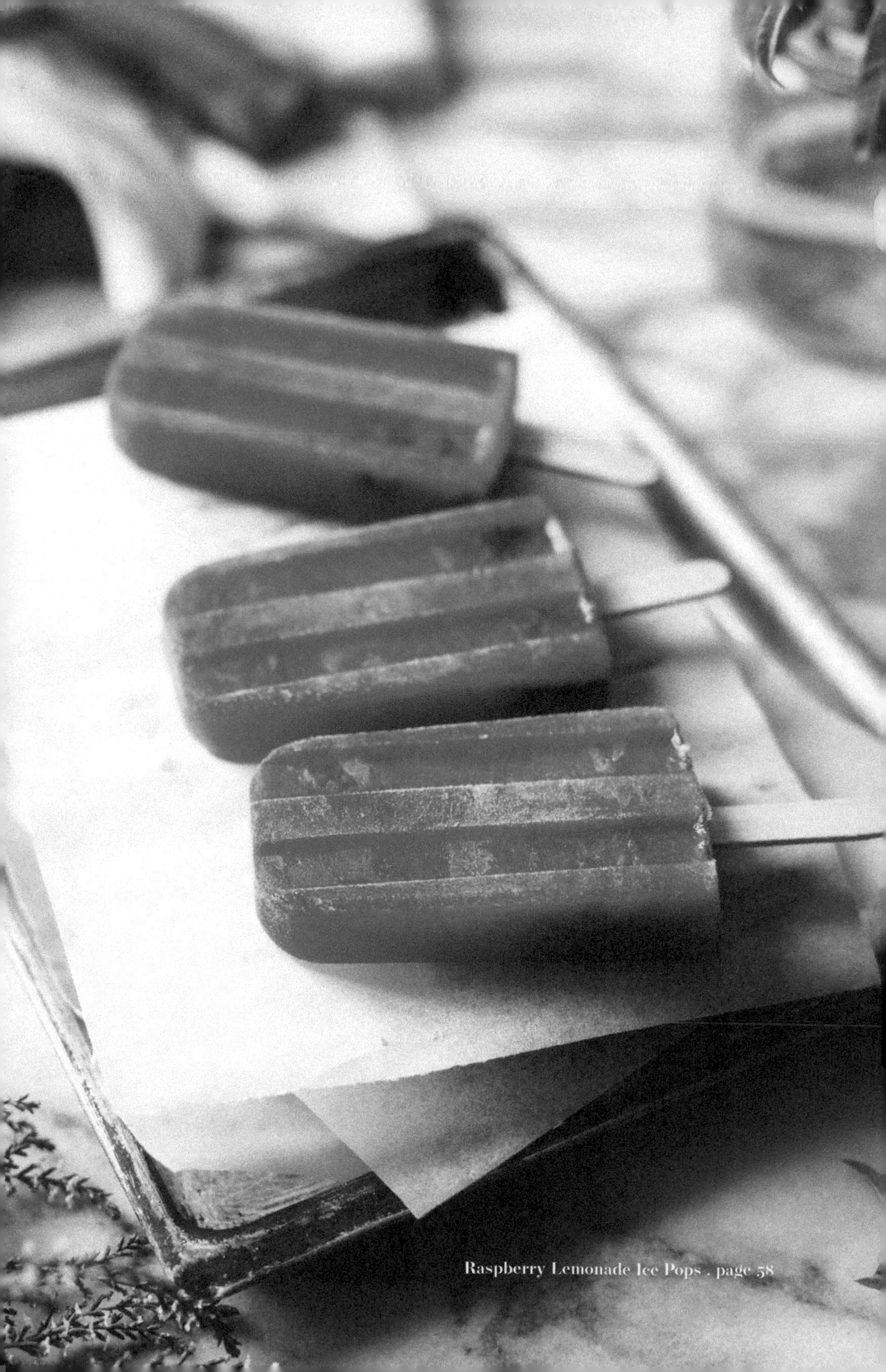

Raspberry Lemonade Ice Pops, page 58

The Essential

DIET FOR DIVERTICULITIS

A 3-Stage Nutrition Guide to Manage and Prevent Flare-Ups

KARYN SUNOHARA, RD

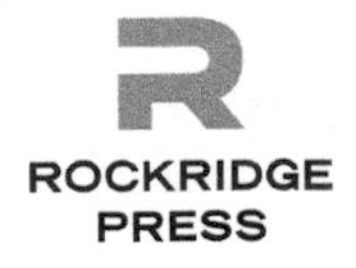

For general information on our other products and services or to obtain technical support, please contact our Customer Care Department within the United States at (866) 744-2665, or outside the United States at (510) 253-0500.

Rockridge Press publishes its books in a variety of electronic and print formats. Some content that appears in print may not be available in electronic books, and vice versa.

Interior and Cover Designer: Monica Cheng
Art Producer: Hannah Dickerson
Editor: Reina Glenn
Production Editor: Nora Milman

Photography © 2020 Helene Dujardin, food styling by Anna Hampton, cover; Illustrations © 2020 Kelsey Garrity-Riley, pp. VIII, 4, 5, 25, 50; StockFood/The Picture Pantry, pp. II, VI, 16; Shutterstock/Justyna Pankowska, p. 2; Stocksy/Ali Harper, p. 26; StockFood/Bauer Syndication, p. 52; Stocksy/Cameron Whitman, p. 62; Stocksy/Ina Peters, p. 90.

Author photo courtesy of © Ronnel Chua

Cover: Chicken and Rice Soup, page 73

ISBN: Print 978-1-64739-414-1 | eBook 978-1-64739-415-8

R1

Contents

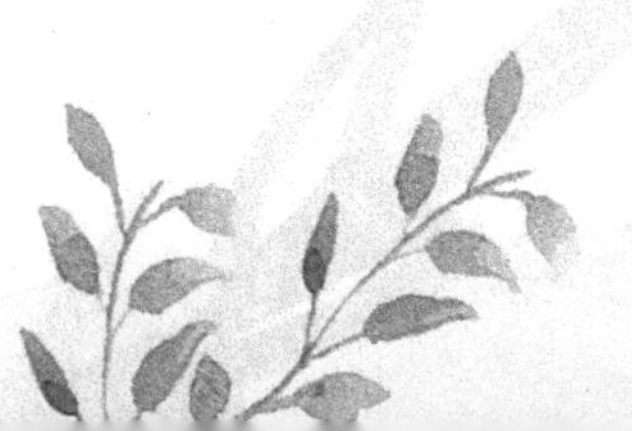

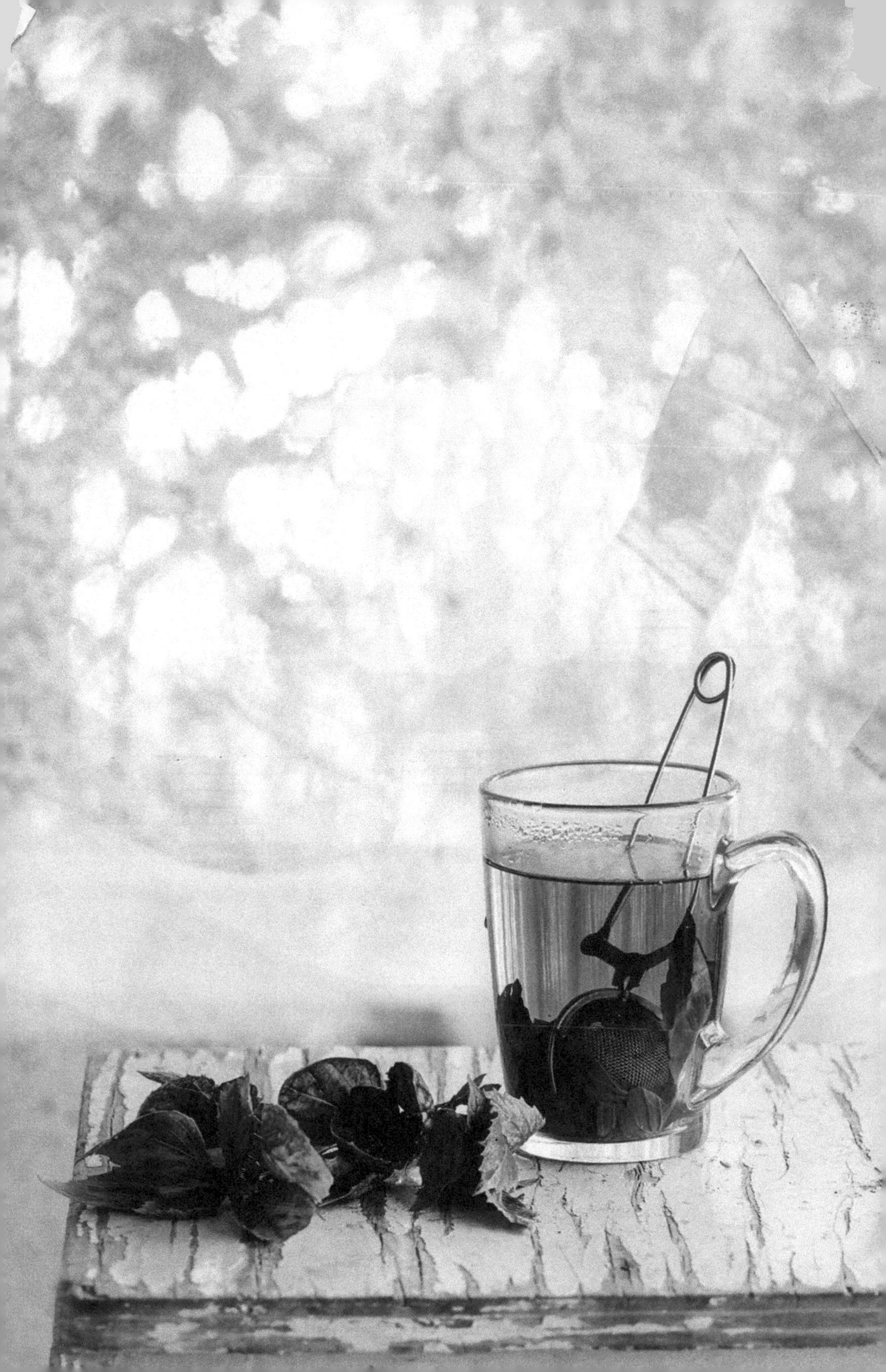

Introduction

A diagnosis of any kind can be overwhelming, but intestinal issues are particularly difficult to manage. Our brains and digestive systems are highly connected, creating innumerable factors that can lead to changes in bowel habits, abdominal pain, and discomfort. Plus, the symptoms are easy to misinterpret—who among us hasn't had a digestive issue after an overly rich meal or a stressful week at work? Many confuse the initial stages of diverticulitis with a stomach bug or food poisoning.

My diverticulitis patients have reported feeling debilitated due to both the symptoms they experience and the lack of information surrounding the condition. While the Internet contains copious information at the click of a button, trying to decipher what intestinal health information is medically sound can feel impossible.

That's why I wrote this book—to provide you the most current, medically accurate information you may not have found elsewhere. During my time in primary care, one of the most common areas I helped patients with was digestive disorders. I've counseled patients after diagnoses of irritable bowel syndrome, inflammatory bowel disease, celiac disease, colon cancer, diverticular disease, and other functional gut disorders. Because of that work, I have developed and facilitated digestive health group classes as well as general healthy eating classes with a focus on healthy lifestyle changes. These days, I work in several different facets of nutrition, including primary care, private practice with an amazing team of registered dietitians at Ignite Nutrition Inc., and my own private practice, For the LOVE of FOOD, where I focus on preventive health, digestive disorders, food relationships, family nutrition, and cooking classes.

In this book, you'll find information on the relationship between diverticular disease and food, including how to prevent, manage, and recover from flare-ups, as well as the recipes you'll need to eat your way through the three stages that make up the diverticulitis diet.

The path toward feeling better begins in just a few pages.

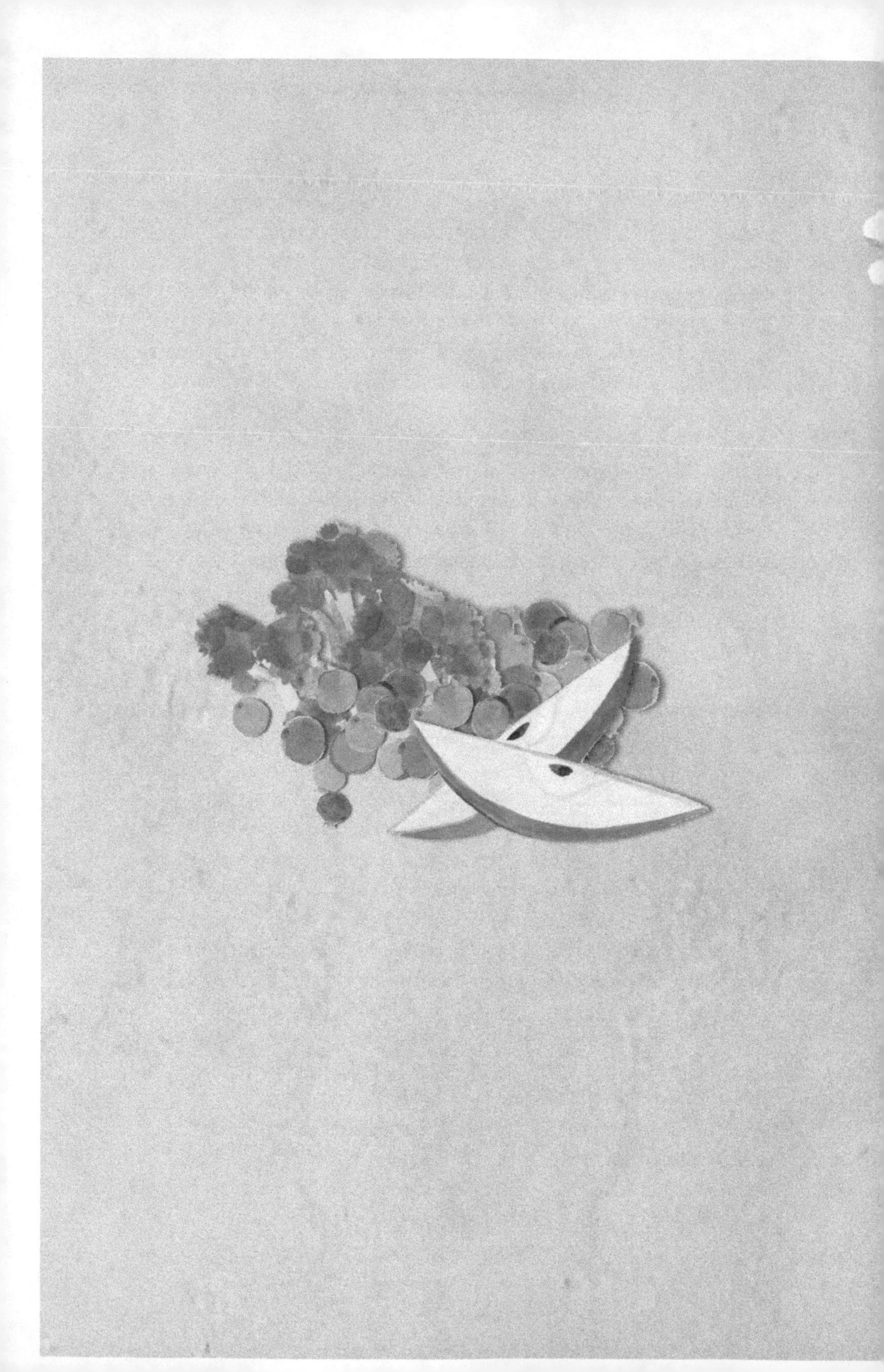

Part I.

Understanding Diverticular Disease

Balsamic Roasted Carrots, page 84

1.

What We Know About Diverticulitis

As you may already know, there are many unanswered questions when it comes to diverticulitis. Through epidemiologic studies, doctors have determined that dietary factors are most likely a cause of the predominance of diverticulitis in North America. However, there is still much to be learned about both the treatment and the effects of digestive disorders. New research findings are appearing every day, but this chapter will cover what we currently know.

What Is Diverticular Disease?

Diverticular disease is one of the most common conditions in Western countries, with particular presence in the United States, Europe, and Australia. According to a 2011 study in the US National Institutes of Health's National Library of Medicine (NIH/NLM), as many as 60 percent of Western people over the age of 70 have diverticular disease, and that number has only grown over the past decade. The disease encompasses three conditions: diverticulosis, diverticulitis, and diverticular bleeding. All of these involve the development of small sacs or pockets in the wall of the colon, called diverticula.

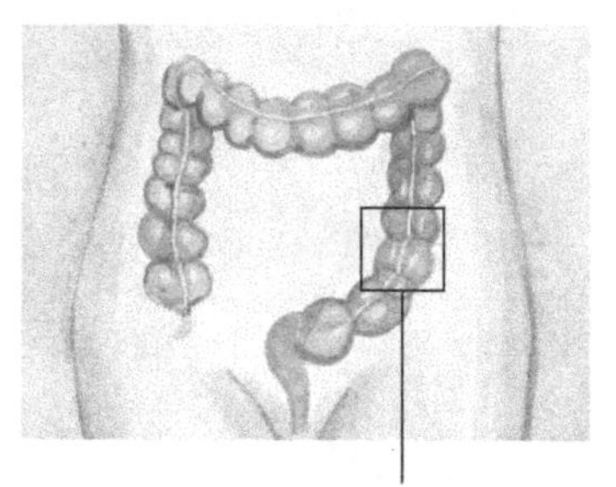

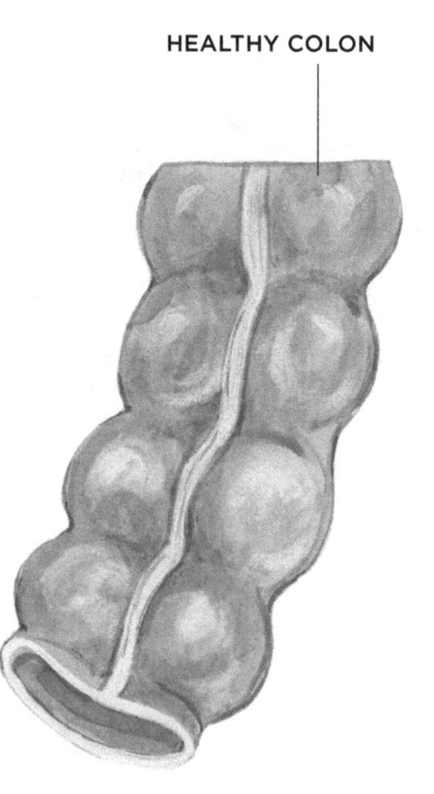

In a healthy individual, the colon is smooth and muscular, but those with diverticular disease have areas where the muscle has weakened (often due to age, because new cells don't rejuvenate as quickly as we get older)—the areas where diverticula are likely to form. From there, the condition can progress through two phases: diverticulosis and diverticulitis.

Diverticulosis

On its own, diverticulosis is not a source of concern—some live a healthy life with no symptoms at all. For others, diverticulosis may cause issues similar to irritable bowel syndrome (IBS), such

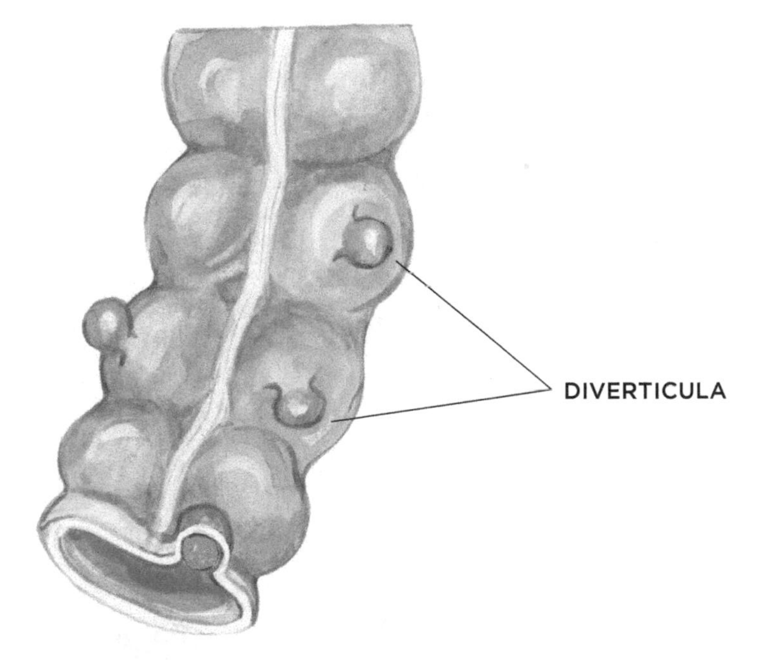

as disruptive changes to regular bowel habits (including diarrhea, constipation, or fluctuation between the two). If stool gets trapped in the pouches (diverticula), it can cause diverticulosis to progress to diverticulitis. Approximately 15 to 20 percent of individuals with diverticulosis will see it turn into diverticulitis, and this rate increases with age.

Diverticulitis

Diverticulitis occurs when the diverticula become inflamed or infected. This can be an acute condition, meaning it's temporary and heals in a short amount of time, or chronic, meaning it's a long-term condition that may heal but never completely goes away. Symptoms of diverticulitis may include diarrhea, abdominal pain (typically in the lower left portion of the abdomen), cramping, constipation, fever, bleeding, and bloating. With diverticulitis, you may experience any combination of these symptoms.

The Progression

There are four stages of diverticulitis progression, which doctors measure using the Hinchey classification method. It's important to understand what stage you're in because if left untreated, diverticulitis can become a chronic issue, leading to bacterial infection or tears in the wall of your colon.

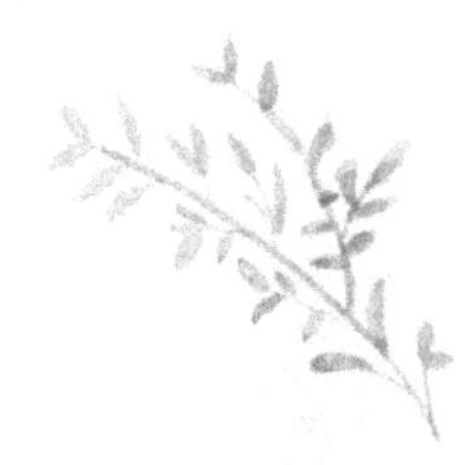

HINCHEY CLASSIFICATION

Stage 0: Mild Clinical Diverticulitis
Symptoms include pain in your lower left abdomen, fever, and elevated white blood cell count. In this stage, you are likely just beginning to experience symptoms and may not have confirmed your diverticulitis diagnosis through digital imagery or surgery.

Stage I: Pericolic Abscess or Phlegmon
The localized inflammation (which is causing the pain in your lower left abdomen) can lead to an abscess, or pocket, in the fat that surrounds the colon. If untreated, it can fill with pus and become infected.

Stage II: Pelvic, Intra-abdominal, or Retroperitoneal Abscess
The abscess has filled with pus or infected fluid, and you may be experiencing abdominal pain, constipation or diarrhea, fever, or vomiting.

Stage III: Generalized Purulent Peritonitis
The abscess is showing signs of bursting, which would drain pus into the abdomen and potentially lead to infection. This stage often requires surgery.

Stage IV: Generalized Fecal Peritonitis
At this stage, the abscess has burst and fecal matter has released into the abdomen, a condition that can cause a dangerous infection, leading to sepsis and even death.

Individuals with uncomplicated diverticulitis (stages 0 to I) are usually able to manage the disease by following a high-fiber diet or, when in an active flare-up, with antibiotics and a clear liquid diet (also known as bowel rest). However, if you have substantial scarring or infected tissue, you may need to have that part of your colon surgically removed to prevent the disease from getting worse.

Think of your colon like a balloon: It can only stretch so much before it pops. Recurring constipation or blockages will stretch your colon in much the same way. As you age, the strength of your colon decreases, which is why diverticulosis disproportionately affects those over the age of 70. The good news? A high-fiber diet can help prevent this added pressure on the colon.

Causes

Digestive disorders are notoriously challenging to narrow down to one cause, and thus doctors have not yet pinpointed a single source for diverticular disease. However, there are a number of factors that may increase your chances of developing it, including a low-fiber diet, consuming red meat more than twice per week, certain medications, obesity, using tobacco products, lack of exercise, increased age, and genetics.

Low Fiber Intake

A low-fiber diet (including high red meat consumption) can lead to constipation, which makes it harder for you to pass stool and puts pressure on your colon. Researchers believe it is this pressure that weakens the bowel tissue and, over time, causes diverticula to form in the wall of the colon.

Medication

Some medications, like steroids and certain pain relievers, can increase your risk of developing diverticulitis. Nonsteroidal anti-inflammatory drugs (NSAIDs) such as aspirin and ibuprofen, in particular, can be very problematic. Consider these statistics from a 2011 NIH/NLM study: Of nearly a thousand people with diverticulitis, those who took aspirin more than twice per week were 25 percent more likely to experience complications than those who were not using NSAIDs. This is because NSAIDs have been proven to damage the lining of the intestinal tract.

Lifestyle Factors

Weight plays a significant role in your likelihood of developing diverticulitis, as excess fat stored in the abdominal cavity causes increased pressure on the colon and raises your risk of developing diverticula. Studies have shown that smokers are also at a higher risk of diverticular disease because smoking has been shown to raise your chances of perforations (tiny tears in the lining of the bowel that weaken the tissues). Finally, decreased or low movement (less than 30 minutes of exercise per day) can lead to constipation, a huge contributor to diverticulitis development. Regular physical activity can help prevent diverticulitis by keeping food moving through your digestive track.

Age

As you get older, the muscles in your colon weaken, increasing your likelihood of developing diverticular disease. In Western countries, it is estimated that 10 percent of people over age 40, and 50 percent of people over age 60, will be diagnosed with diverticulosis. That number keeps climbing the older you get.

Genetics

Unfortunately, sometimes your chances of developing diverticular disease live in your DNA, no matter your diet or lifestyle. Though there is no published literature that has been able to identify a genetic link to diverticular disease, observational data does suggest the relationship, as there are differences in where the diverticula form depending on ethnicity. In Western countries, diverticula most commonly form in the descending parts of the colon (see diagram on page 5), while in Asian countries, diverticula occur primarily in the ascending colon. These differences have led researchers to believe there could be genetic factors affecting the origin of diverticulitis.

Signs and Symptoms

The symptoms of diverticulosis and diverticulitis may differ for each person, from none to all of the following signs, so use this list as a guideline.

Diverticulosis

- Bloating
- Fluctuating bowel habits
- Constipation
- Diarrhea
- Pain and cramping

Diverticulitis

- Nausea or vomiting
- Chills and fever
- Pain in the lower left portion of the abdomen
- Rectal bleeding
- Black or maroon-colored stool

Keep track of your symptoms with a free food and symptoms diary, available as a companion to this book at http://callistomediabooks.com/TheEssentialDietforDiverticulitis. If the fever, vomiting, or rectal bleeding continue throughout the day or get worse, seek medical attention immediately. Your doctor may recommend a colonoscopy to rule out inflammatory bowel disease or colon cancer.

Identifying and Managing Flare-Ups

A flare-up from diverticulitis occurs when the diverticula become inflamed or infected, leading to nausea, vomiting, chills, fever, abdominal pain, rectal bleeding, or blood in your stool. If you've experienced flare-ups before, you know that this can be a debilitating time, but there are ways to speed up your recovery.

First, a low-residue (or low-fiber) diet can help slow down your bowel habits. That may sound counterintuitive given the risk of constipation, but during a flare-up, you want to put your colon through the least amount of movement possible to reduce the inflammation of the diverticula. In extreme cases, you may need to resort to a clear fluid diet for a few days to completely halt all bowel movement. When your symptoms begin to subside, you can progress to a low-residue diet and then on to a high-fiber diet again once you've made it through the flare-up. Be sure to increase your fiber intake slowly and steadily—the goal is to gradually bulk up the stool so you can pass it without straining. When you're through the flare-up, focus on eating a high-fiber diet, exercising for at least 30 minutes per day, and drinking lots of water to help prevent future flare-ups. See pages 27–49 for meal plans that cover each of these stages.

Studies show that approximately 20 percent of patients who have one diverticulitis flare-up will have another within five years, so don't delay in seeing your doctor when you experience them. This period may be painful, but it's the easiest time for doctors to diagnose your diverticulitis. Continuous flare-ups may cause damage to the colon that requires surgery, which is why managing and preventing them is paramount. Use the following timeline to track your flare-up progression. You'll know it's okay to move on to the next stage of your diet when the pain subsides and your bowel movements normalize with no pain or straining.

Treatment Options

By now you know that changing your diet is one of the best preventive measures you can take to avoid further flare-ups. However, there are nondietary steps to take in combination with changes to your current eating habits. Keep in mind that you should always consult your doctor before pursuing any new tactics that may affect your digestive and overall health.

Probiotics

These supplements contain certain strains of bacteria that have been proven to alleviate abdominal pain, bloating, constipation, and diarrhea and can help improve the function of your gut's natural microorganisms. However, it's important to talk to your doctor when choosing a probiotic, as they're not all made the same. For example, most probiotics contain lactose, which is not a good choice if you're sensitive to dairy. Studies on diverticulitis and probiotics have shown promising outcomes, but more research is needed before the relationship is considered clinically significant.

Prebiotics

Prebiotics are a type of dietary fiber that helps feed healthy bacteria in the large intestine. They occur naturally in many foods, such as bananas, barley, apples, leeks, asparagus, chicory, Jerusalem artichokes, garlic, onions, wheat, oats, flaxseed, oat bran, jicama root, seaweed, and soybeans.

Antibiotics

Though antibiotics have often been used to help reduce pain, infection, and fever in moderate to severe cases of diverticulitis, newer research is leaning toward reducing the length of antibiotic usage. A 2014 study published in *Drug, Healthcare and Patient Safety* comparing four- and seven-day courses of antibiotics found that they had equivalent outcomes, implying that diverticulitis sufferers do not need to be on antibiotics for extended periods of time.

Surgery

If you've had many flare-ups, the damage to your colon may be too advanced to see improvement from medication or diet, and your doctor may recommend surgery to remove the affected area. There are a few options they may consider:

Simple colostomy: During this procedure, the surgeon pulls a small section of the colon out through an incision in the abdomen and attaches a pouch that will collect waste. This allows your bowel an extended period to heal without any stool moving through it. If your colon heals well from the surgery, the colostomy may be only temporary.

Bowel resection: This is the removal of the infected part of the colon, followed by reconnection of the bowel. The surgeon cuts away the damaged area and reconnects the intestine, sometimes to the rectum.

Both a bowel resection and a simple colostomy can be done open or closed.

Open: The surgeon makes a 6- to 8-inch incision in your abdomen to see a full view of the affected digestive tract.

Closed (or laparoscopic): The surgeon makes a very small incision (typically less than 1 centimeter) and inserts a small tube with a camera and surgical instruments through it to perform the surgery.

Lifestyle Changes

One reason diverticulitis may be so common in North America is because many North Americans eat a fairly low-fiber diet and lead more sedentary lifestyles. Diverticulitis is unheard of in Africa or the Middle East, where the typical diet relies heavily on high-fiber foods such as whole grains and legumes. It's no surprise then that increasing your fiber intake (when you are not experiencing a flare-up) is a good way to keep diverticulitis symptoms at bay. But it's not the only lifestyle change that can help.

Physical Activity

For adults age 18 or older, doctors recommend getting at least 150 minutes of moderate to vigorous aerobic physical activity per week, in increments of at least 10 minutes at a time. They also suggest including muscle- and bone-strengthening exercises one to two days per week. Not only does regular physical activity help reduce your weight and increase muscle formation, it has proven to be beneficial in helping the bowels move stool through the body.

Hydration

As you increase your fiber intake, it's also important to stay hydrated to aid digestion. The average recommended water consumption per day is 2 to 2½ liters for women and 2½ to 3 liters for men. Increasing your fluid intake will help prevent dehydration, which can be a problem if you are having frequent loose bowel movements. It also protects against constipation, which is a side effect of increased fiber without proper hydration.

Losing Weight

Obesity has been shown to increase complications with diverticulitis, namely because of its link to chronic inflammation. It also can contribute to your risk of developing several other digestive diseases, such as liver scarring (cirrhosis), gallstone disease, gastroesophageal reflux disease (GERD), colon cancer, esophageal cancer, and pancreatic cancer. But there's good news: Losing just 5 to 10 percent of your body weight can decrease your risk of complications.

Quitting Tobacco Products

Along with increasing your risk of lung cancer, tobacco products have been shown to decrease blood flow to vital organs, which can cause tissues to die and raise your risk for infection. But quitting can have immediate benefits: Studies have shown that the stomach and lining of the small intestine will return to normal within a few hours of quitting tobacco use. Foregoing tobacco products for the long term can reverse some of the more serious harmful effects tobacco has on the digestive system as well.

Oat Bars with Raspberry
Chia Jam . page 135

2.

Eating Your Way to Intestinal Health

In this chapter, we will explore the ins and outs of fiber and its role in your diverticulitis journey. You will also find an in-depth explanation of how to manage your symptoms through your diet, including what types of foods to eat when. Then I'll provide strategies to help during a flare-up and ways to prevent them in the future. Let's get started.

Fiber—Friend or Foe?

A very common question for people with diverticulitis is whether fiber is considered beneficial or harmful. This confusion makes sense because at certain points you need to avoid it and at other times you need to embrace it. The short answer? It depends on your symptoms.

Before we talk about how fiber affects diverticulitis, it's first important to know that not all fiber is made the same. There are two different types, each with a different purpose.

Soluble Fiber

When it comes into contact with water, soluble fiber turns into a gel and dissolves. This type of fiber can help lower both cholesterol and blood glucose because it slows down your body's absorption of cholesterol and sugar during digestion. This slowing helps you feel full for longer after you eat and prevents constipation. You can find soluble fiber in apples, applesauce, oatmeal, oat bran, avocados, barley, pears, sweet potatoes, legumes, and potatoes. Another, newer type of soluble fiber is inulin, a tasteless fiber product that has recently been added to foods such as yogurt, cereal, pasta, granola bars, and bread products. Natural sources of inulin include bananas, onions, garlic, asparagus, and chicory root.

Insoluble Fiber

Insoluble fiber does not dissolve in water, which makes it helpful in adding bulk to the stool. This allows stool to move through the digestive tract more quickly, creating a laxative effect that combats constipation. Insoluble fiber helps reduce the risk of colon cancer and heart disease. Sources of insoluble fiber are wheat bran, corn bran, whole grains, nuts, and all fruits and vegetables.

The Diet Stages

There are three main stages to the diverticulitis diet: managing an active flare-up, recovering from it, and preventing it in the future. Throughout each stage, **it is crucial that you listen to your body**

and make diet adjustments slowly, adding one or two new foods at a time while closely monitoring your symptoms.

During a Flare-Up: Clear Fluids

If your flare-up symptoms are extreme, you may need to give your bowel a period of rest. A clear fluid diet will help your body recuperate because it may be temporarily unable to tolerate any solid foods. Keep in mind that this is not meant to be a long-term diet—you should follow it for only a couple of days. Restricting yourself to a clear fluid diet for any length of time may cause you to feel weak, light-headed, fatigued, and hungry. Other symptoms include excessive weight loss, muscle wasting, and depletion of vitamins and minerals. These symptoms occur because it's very difficult to meet the body's daily caloric requirements for protein, carbohydrates, and fat through a clear fluid diet. In order to provide your body with enough energy, you need to consume at least 200 grams of carbohydrates throughout the day. If you have blood sugar challenges such as low blood sugar or diabetes, you may want to monitor your blood sugars during this stage.

The Clear Fluids Diet Breakdown

EAT THIS	AVOID THAT
Boost clear or Boost juice	Any solid foods
Clear, fat-free broth	Condiments of any kind
Coffee or tea with no milk products or creamers	Fruit skins, seeds, or pulp
Gelatin Pulp-free juice	Milk and milk alternative
Pedialyte	Peanut butter
Pulp-free fruit ice pops	Smoothies
Soda	Yogurt drinks
Sports drinks	

After a Flare-Up: Low-Residue Foods

A low-residue (or low-fiber) diet acts as the reintroduction phase, after your flare-up symptoms have mostly passed but before your body is ready for high-fiber foods. "Residue" is the indigestible fiber that passes through the large intestine and then is excreted as stool. The goal of this diet is to reduce the number of bowel

The Low-Residue Diet Breakdown

EAT THIS

Asparagus tips (cooked)

Bananas

Beets (cooked)

Butter

Cantaloupe

Carrots (cooked)

Eggplant (cooked)

Eggs

Fish

Green onions (cooked)

Honeydew melon

Jelly (seedless)

Margarine

Mayonnaise

Meal replacement nutritional drinks

Mushrooms (cooked)

Oil

Peaches (peeled and cooked)

Pears (peeled and cooked)

Peas (cooked)

Potatoes (peeled and mashed)

Poultry

Refined (white) **flour products: noodles, rice, couscous, tortillas, bread, etc.**

Refined cereals: Rice Krispies, Cheerios, cornflakes, instant oatmeal, Cream of Wheat

Salad dressing of any type

Smooth nut butters (peanut, almond)

Spinach (cooked)

Squash (peeled and well-cooked)

Sweet potatoes (peeled and well-cooked)

Watermelon

Yams (peeled and well-cooked)

Yogurt drinks

movements you have, which will in turn decrease the pain associated with the flare-up. Like the clear fluid stage, the low-residue diet is not meant to be a long-term lifestyle. You should only follow it while you are recovering from inflammation and flare-up pain. Once the pain subsides, you can start introducing more high-fiber foods, working your way up to a high-fiber diet.

AVOID THAT

Avocados

Beans

Berries with seeds (such as strawberries or raspberries)

Broccoli

Brussels sprouts

Cabbage

Cauliflower

Cherries

Chickpeas

Corn

Crunchy nut butters

Dried fruit

Fried fruits

Fruit seeds or skins

Grapefruit (raw)

Kale

Kiwi

Lentils

Mango (raw)

Onions

Oranges (raw)

Pickles or relish

Pineapple (raw)

Popcorn

Raw vegetables of any kind

Red meat

String beans

Whole nuts or seeds

Whole-grain or whole-wheat cereal, bread, pasta, rice, crackers, or bagels

Flare-Up Prevention: High-Fiber Foods

This final stage of the diverticulitis diet is the maintenance and prevention phase—in other words, your normal eating routine. When you're not suffering or recovering from a flare-up, a high-fiber diet can protect against the development of diverticula by keeping bowel movements regular and easy. However, you do not want to go from

The High-Fiber Diet Breakdown

EAT THIS	AVOID THAT
Avocados	**Refined white flour or white rice products**
Barley	**Red meat** (more than 2 servings per week)
Beans	
Berries (especially blackberries and raspberries)	
Broccoli	
Brown rice	
Bulgur	
Cauliflower	
Cereal	
Chia seeds	
Chickpeas	
Crunchy nut butters	
Flax	
Hemp seeds	**Note:** *Though you are still allowed to eat fish and poultry on the high-fiber diet, these are not high-fiber proteins, so they are not included in this chart.*
Kiwi	
Lentils	
Pears	
Raw vegetables	
Whole-grain pastas, bread, crackers, and bran cereal	
Wild rice	

a low-fiber diet straight to a high-fiber diet, as this can damage your colon. **Slow and steady is the rule when it comes to fiber increase**: Aim to increase your fiber intake by 2 to 4 grams per week until you reach the recommended amount for your age and biology. Keep in mind that as you increase your fiber, you also need to increase your water intake to help move the fiber through your intestinal tract.

Recommended Daily Doses of Fiber and Water

Recommended Fiber Intake:

Men age 19 to 50 = 38 grams per day
Men age 50+ = 30 grams per day
Women age 19 to 50 = 25 grams per day
Women age 50+ = 21 grams per day

Recommended Water Intake:

Men age 19+ = 12 cups (about 3 liters) per day
Women age 19+ = 9 cups (about 2 liters) per day

Nuts, Seeds, and Popcorn

It was long thought that diverticulitis sufferers should avoid nuts, seeds, and popcorn for fear of these foods getting caught in the diverticula and causing an infection. However, a 2009 survey of over 45,000 health professionals reported that diverticulitis was not associated with the ingestion of corn, popcorn, nuts, or seeds. In fact, the survey found that increased intake of these foods actually lowered the risk of diverticulitis because most nuts, seeds, corn, and popcorn are high sources of fiber.

Trigger Foods

No matter what stage of the diet you're in, there may be some foods that are problematic for you. These foods are typically high in fat or sugar, spicy, caffeinated, or fried. Keeping a food and symptoms diary is one way to help identify possible trigger foods for your body. You can download one for free as a companion to this book by visiting http://callistomediabooks.com/TheEssentialDietforDiverticulitis. Remember that everybody reacts differently to food, so a trigger for you may not affect someone else with diverticulitis, and vice versa. Here are some common examples of trigger foods.

High-FODMAP Foods

FODMAP stands for "fermentable oligosaccharides, disaccharides, monosaccharides, and polyols." These carbohydrates don't get absorbed by the small intestine and end up fermenting in your colon, creating gas and contributing to intestinal issues such as bloating, pain, diarrhea, and constipation. Because high-FODMAP foods have been shown to increase pressure in the colon, researchers are currently studying whether going on a low-FODMAP diet temporarily will help identify diverticulitis triggers. Some examples of high-FODMAP food triggers include wheat, garlic, onions, peaches, apples, soy, lactose, and beans. There's no proven correlation as of yet—more research is needed before doctors can recommend a low-FODMAP diet for diverticulitis sufferers.

High-Fat Foods

Fat takes the body approximately 40 hours to digest and excrete, a number that only goes up if you suffer from diverticular disease. This means that consuming high-fat foods is particularly harmful to your digestion. More generally, high-fat foods increase your risk of obesity, which studies have linked to increased risk for and complications with diverticular disease.

Too Much Fiber

Though it seems contradictory, some studies suggest that too much fiber can cause constipation if not matched with lots of water, which may in turn worsen diverticulitis symptoms. Everyone's body has a different tolerance for fiber, so use the recommended fiber and fluid intakes as a guide and keep track of your symptoms, adjusting as necessary to suit your specific biology.

The Balanced Plate

Think of the balanced plate as an approach to healthy eating instead of a diet. When you're not experiencing or recovering from a flare-up, aim for this breakdown: ½ of the plate is made up of vegetables, ¼ is high-fiber starch, and ¼ is lean protein. There is no need to try to figure out the calories or macronutrients in the food—simply aim for these ratios when you're at a family dinner or buffet. For example, a balanced dinner could look like 4 ounces of chicken breast, ½ cup cooked brown rice, and 1 cup steamed vegetables.

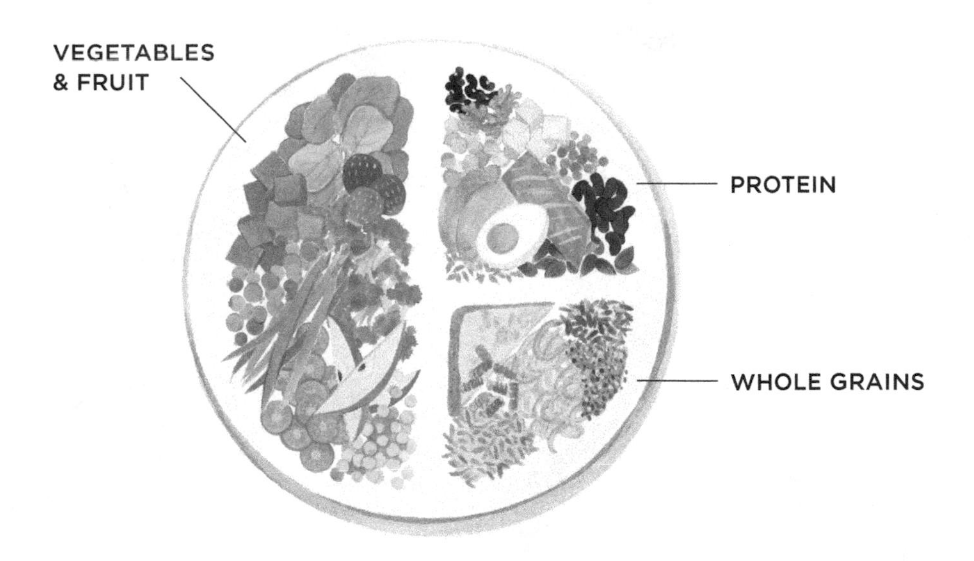

Overnight Steel-Cut Oats . page 97

3.

The Meal Plans

When you're coping with a new medical diagnosis, figuring out what to eat can be challenging. I've created the following meal plans as a guide to help you through each stage of the diverticulitis diet, including shopping lists to save you time at the store. Remember to consult your doctor before progressing through each diet stage to make sure your body is ready for a fiber increase.

During a Flare-Up

If your flare-up symptoms are extreme, a clear fluid diet will allow your bowels a short period of rest. Short is the key word here—**you should not be on a clear fluid diet for more than three days, and only if it's recommended by your doctor**. A prolonged period on this diet can lead to weight loss, weakness, muscle loss, dizziness, and malnutrition.

Clear Fluids

	BREAKFAST	LUNCH	DINNER
Day 1	Apple-Cinnamon Tea *(page 54)*	Homemade Chicken Stock *(page 61)*	Homemade Orange Gelatin *(page 57)*
Day 2	Blueberry Green Tea *(page 55)*	Homemade Beef Stock *(page 60)*	Raspberry Lemonade Ice Pops *(page 58)*
Day 3	Apple-Cinnamon Tea *(page 54)*	Citrus Sports Drink *(page 56)*	Tropical Ice Pops *(page 59)*

Shopping List: Clear Fluids

FREEZER SECTION

Blueberries, frozen (4 ounces)
Raspberries, frozen (24 ounces)

PRODUCE

Apples, Honey Crisp, Fuji, Granny Smith, or Gala (4)
Carrots (8)
Celery (1 head)
Garlic (1 bulb)
Lemon juice
Onions, white or Spanish (2)
Oranges, large (20)

MEAT

Beef bones, with marrow if possible (2 pounds)
Chicken carcass (2 pounds)

BAKING AISLE

Gelatin, unflavored
Honey
Maple syrup

HERBS AND SPICES

Bay leaves
Cinnamon sticks (6)
Peppercorns, black
Sage, dried
Salt
Sea salt
Thyme, dried

OTHER

Coconut water (36 ounces)
Earl Grey tea, caffeinated or decaffeinated
Green tea, caffeinated or decaffeinated

After a Flare-Up

As you recover from a flare-up, it's important to slowly transition to a low-residue diet. The recipes in this meal plan are listed from lowest to highest fiber levels to ensure your body has time to get used to the increasing fiber intake. The order of the recipes is carefully selected to ensure that you cook once and eat twice—wisely using leftovers to prevent you from having to cook every meal from scratch.

Week 1: Low-Residue

	BREAKFAST	LUNCH	DINNER
Day 1	Greek Yogurt Banana Pancakes *(page 68)*	Chicken and Rice Soup *(page 73)*	Salmon Cakes *(page 80)*
Day 2	Avocado Eggs *(page 69)*	Leftover Salmon Cakes	Pad Thai *(page 78)*
Day 3	Peach Scones *(page 66)*	Leftover Pad Thai	One-Pot Chicken and Orzo *(page 75)*
Day 4	Apple-Cinnamon Muffins *(page 65)*	Leftover One-Pot Chicken and Orzo	Chicken and Rice Soup *(page 73)*
Day 5	Avocado Eggs *(page 69)*	Panzanella Salad *(page 82)*	Leftover Chicken and Rice Soup
Day 6	Strawberry Cheesecake Smoothie *(page 64)*	Salmon Cakes *(page 80)*	Spinach, Mushroom, and Bacon Quiche *(page 70)*
Day 7	Leftover Apple-Cinnamon Muffins	Leftover Spinach, Mushroom, and Bacon Quiche	Cod en Papillote *(page 81)*

Week 1 Shopping List: Low-Residue

CANNED GOODS

Applesauce, unsweetened
Chicken stock (5 quarts)
Peaches, canned, packed in water (1 [14.5-ounce] can)

CONDIMENTS AND SAUCES

Dijon mustard
Fish sauce
Hot sauce
Rice vinegar
Soy sauce
Sriracha or hot chili paste
Tamarind paste (or brown sugar and lime juice)

DAIRY AND EGGS

Bocconcini (mozzarella) balls (4 ounces)
Butter or margarine
Cheddar cheese, shredded (8 ounces)
Cheese of choice, shredded (8 ounces)
Cottage cheese (8 ounces)
Eggs, large
Greek yogurt, plain
Milk
Parmesan cheese, grated (4 ounces)

FREEZER SECTION

Peas and carrots, mixed, frozen
Pie shell, 9-inch premade (1)
Spinach, frozen (1 [10-ounce] package)
Strawberries, frozen (16 ounces)

PRODUCE

Apples, Honey Crisp, Fuji, Granny Smith, or Gala (2)
Asparagus (1 bunch)
Avocados, ripe (2)
Banana (1)
Basil, fresh (1 bunch)
Bean sprouts (8 ounces)
Bell peppers, red (2)
Carrots (1 pound)
Celery (1 head)
Chives (1 bunch)
Cilantro, fresh (optional) (1 bunch)
Cucumber, English (1)
Garlic (1 bulb)
Green onions (6)
Lemon (1)
Lemon juice

Lime (1)
Mushrooms (4 ounces)
Onion, red (1) or shallots (2)
Onion, white or Spanish (1)
Potatoes, Yukon Gold (2)
Tomatoes, Roma (4)

MEAT AND FISH

Bacon or precooked bacon bits
Chicken (20 ounces)
Cod, boneless, skinless (4 [5-ounce] fillets)
Salmon, boneless, skinless (½ pound)
Shrimp, large, peeled and deveined (1 pound)

GRAINS AND STARCHES

Bread crumbs
Burger buns, white (6)
French bread or baguette, white, day-old (1)
Orzo pasta
Rice, jasmine
Rice noodles, flat (10 ounces)

BAKING AISLE

Baking powder
Baking soda
Flour, all-purpose
Honey
Maple syrup
Oil, canola
Oil, olive
Oil, peanut
Oil, vegetable
Sugar
Vanilla extract
Vinegar, balsamic

HERBS AND SPICES

Bay leaf
Cinnamon, ground
Freshly ground black pepper
Garlic powder
Onion powder
Paprika
Salt

Week 2: Low-Residue

	BREAKFAST	LUNCH	DINNER
Day 1	Apple-Cinnamon Muffins *(page 65)*	Leftover Cod en Papillote *(from Week 1)*	Creamy Mushroom Soup *(page 72)*
Day 2	Avocado Eggs *(page 69)*	Leftover Creamy Mushroom Soup	Shrimp Curry *(page 76)*
Day 3	Peach Scones *(page 66)*	Leftover Shrimp Curry	Spinach, Mushroom, and Bacon Quiche *(page 70)*
Day 4	Leftover Apple-Cinnamon Muffins	Panzanella Salad *(page 82)*	One-Pot Chicken and Orzo *(page 75)*
Day 5	Peach Scones *(page 66)*	Leftover One-Pot Chicken and Orzo	Pad Thai *(page 78)*
Day 6	Avocado Eggs *(page 69)*	Leftover Pad Thai	Cod en Papillote *(page 81)*
Day 7	Greek Yogurt Banana Pancakes *(page 68)*	Leftover Cod en Papillote	Creamy Mushroom Soup *(page 72)*

Week 2 Shopping List: Low-Residue

CANNED GOODS

Applesauce, unsweetened
Chicken stock (1 quart)
Coconut milk, unsweetened (1 [13½-ounce] can)
Peaches, canned, packed in water (1 [14.5-ounce] can)
Tomato paste (1 [13-ounce] can)
Vegetable broth

CONDIMENTS AND SAUCES

Balsamic vinegar
Fish sauce
Rice vinegar
Soy sauce
Sriracha or hot chili paste
Tamarind paste (or brown sugar and lime juice)

DAIRY AND EGGS

Bocconcini (mozzarella) balls (4 ounces)
Butter or margarine
Cheddar cheese, shredded (8 ounces)
Cheese of choice, shredded (8 ounces)
Eggs, large
Greek yogurt, plain
Milk
Parmesan cheese, grated (4 ounces)
Whipping cream

FREEZER SECTION

Peas and carrots, mixed, frozen
Pie shell, 9-inch premade (1)
Spinach, frozen (1 [10-ounce] package)

PRODUCE

Apples, Honey Crisp, Fuji, Granny Smith, or Gala (2)
Asparagus (1 bunch)
Avocados, ripe (2)
Banana (1)
Basil, fresh (1 bunch)
Bean sprouts (8 ounces)
Bell peppers, red (2)
Carrots (2)
Cilantro, fresh (optional) (1 bunch)
Cucumber, English (1)
Garlic (1 bulb)
Green onions (6)
Lemon (1)
Lime (1)
Lime juice
Mushrooms, button (24 ounces)

Mushrooms (4 ounces)
Mushrooms, portabella (2)
Onion, red (1) or shallots (2)
Onions, white or Spanish (2)
Potatoes, Yukon Gold (2)
Tomatoes, Roma (4)

MEAT AND FISH

Bacon or precooked bacon bits
Chicken (8 ounces)
Cod, boneless, skinless (4 [5-ounce] fillets)
Shrimp, large, peeled and deveined (2 pounds)

GRAINS AND STARCHES

French bread or baguette, white, day-old (1)
Rice, jasmine
Rice noodles, flat (10 ounces)
Orzo pasta

BAKING AISLE

Baking powder
Baking soda
Flour, all-purpose
Honey
Maple syrup
Oil, canola
Oil, olive
Oil, peanut
Oil, vegetable
Sugar
Vanilla extract

HERBS AND SPICES

Cinnamon, ground
Curry paste, yellow
Freshly ground black pepper
Garlic powder
Ginger, ground
Onion powder
Salt
Thyme, dried

OTHER

White wine, pinot grigio or sauvignon blanc

Flare-Up Prevention

This stage of the diet should make up the majority of your meals when you are not in an active flare-up. I've created a meal plan for four weeks of high-fiber foods, but you should continue eating high-fiber foods for the foreseeable future to prevent flare-ups. This is the best time to keep track of your symptoms, as the foods you eat during this period will affect your ongoing intestinal health. A free food and symptoms diary is available as a companion to this book. Download it at http://callistomediabooks.com/TheEssentialDietforDiverticulitis.

Week 1: High-Fiber

	BREAKFAST	LUNCH	DINNER
Day 1	Strawberry-Banana Breakfast Parfait *(page 94)*	Taco Salad *(page 110)*	Vegetable Stir-Fry *(page 114)*
Day 2	Leftover Strawberry-Banana Breakfast Parfait	Leftover Vegetable Stir-Fry	Minestrone Soup *(page 104)*
Day 3	Apple-Cinnamon Baked Oatmeal Squares *(page 96)*	Leftover Minestrone Soup	Lentil Curry *(page 117)*
Day 4	Leftover Apple-Cinnamon Baked Oatmeal Squares	Leftover Lentil Curry	Jambalaya *(page 108)*
Day 5	Chocolate-Peanut Butter Smoothie Bowls *(page 93)*	Leftover Jambalaya	Farro Risotto *(page 119)*
Day 6	Almond-Orange Cranberry Loaf *(page 99)*	Leftover Farro Risotto	Black Bean Burgers *(page 120)*
Day 7	Leftover Almond-Orange Cranberry Loaf	Santa Fe Cobb Salad *(page 111)*	Stuffed Sweet Potatoes *(page 112)*

Week 1 Shopping List: High-Fiber

CANNED GOODS

Applesauce, unsweetened
Black beans (2 [15½-ounce] cans)
Chicken stock (1 quart)
Chickpeas (1 [15½-ounce] can)
Coconut milk
Corn, roasted, canned (8 ounces)
Kidney beans (1 [15-ounce] can)
Orange juice
Pineapple or orange juice
Tomato paste (1 [6-ounce] can plus 1 tablespoon)
Tomatoes, crushed (1 [15-ounce] can)
Tomatoes, diced (1 [28-ounce] can)
Vegetable stock (8½ cups)

CONDIMENTS AND SAUCES

Dijon mustard
Hot sauce
Peanut butter
Salad dressing, ranch, blue cheese, or chipotle ranch
Salsa
Sesame oil
Soy sauce
Tahini

DAIRY AND EGGS

Butter or margarine
Eggs, large
Feta cheese, crumbled (4 ounces)
Goat cheese, crumbled (4 ounces)
Greek yogurt, plain
Milk
Parmesan cheese, grated (2 ounces)
Sour cream or plain Greek yogurt
Whipping cream

FREEZER SECTION

Carrots and green beans, mixed, frozen
Edamame, shelled, frozen
Peas and carrots, mixed, frozen

PRODUCE

Apples, Honey Crisp, Fuji, Granny Smith, or Gala (2)
Avocados (3)
Bananas (4)
Bell peppers, green (3)
Bell peppers, red (4)
Broccoli florets (1 head)
Carrots (2)
Cauliflower florets (1 head)
Celery (1 head)
Cucumber, English (1)
Garlic (1 bulb)
Green onions (2 bunches)
Lemon juice
Lettuce, romaine (2 large heads)
Lime juice
Mushrooms, button (8 ounces)
Onion, red (1)
Onions, white or Spanish (4)
Orange (1)
Spinach (1 pound)
Strawberries (16 ounces)
Sugar snap peas (8 ounces)
Sweet potatoes, medium (4)
Tomatoes, cherry (12 ounces)
Tomatoes, Roma (7)
Zucchini (1)

MEAT AND FISH

Bacon
Chicken breast, boneless, skinless (1)
Chicken or turkey, lean ground (½ pound)
Shrimp, large, peeled and deveined (½ pound)

GRAINS AND STARCHES

Bread crumbs
Burger buns, whole-wheat (4)
Farro
Lentils, red, dried
Oats or muesli
Oats, rolled
Pasta shells, small, high-fiber
Quinoa
Rice, brown basmati

BAKING AISLE

Almonds, sliced
Baking powder
Baking soda
Chia seeds
Cocoa powder, unsweetened dark
Cornstarch
Cranberries, dried unsweetened
Flaxseed, ground
Flour, whole-wheat
Honey or maple syrup
Pumpkin seeds

- Sugar, brown
- Sugar, granulated
- Vanilla extract
- Vegetable oil

HERBS AND SPICES

- Cajun seasoning
- Cinnamon, ground
- Cumin, ground
- Curry powder
- Freshly ground black pepper
- Garam masala
- Italian seasoning
- Salt
- Taco seasoning

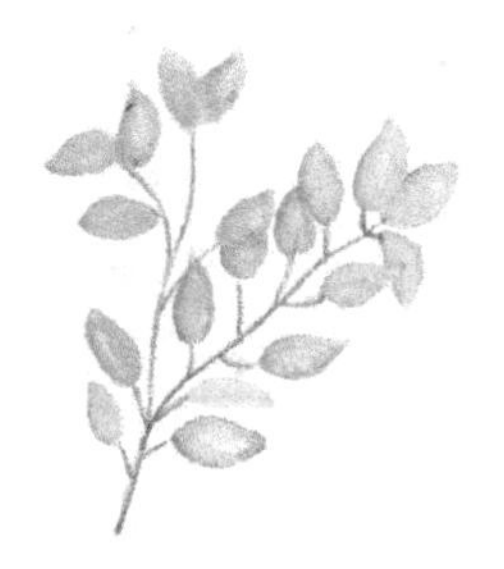

Week 2: High-Fiber

	BREAKFAST	LUNCH	DINNER
Day 1	Chocolate-Peanut Butter Smoothie Bowls *(page 93)*	Leftover Stuffed Sweet Potatoes *(from Week 1)*	Meat Sauce with Lentils *(page 124)*
Day 2	Almond-Orange Cranberry Loaf *(page 99)*	Leftover Meat Sauce with Lentils	Vegetarian Sushi Bowls *(page 115)*
Day 3	Vegetarian Breakfast Burritos *(page 102)*	Leftover Vegetarian Sushi Bowls	High-Fiber Mac and Cheese *(page 116)*
Day 4	Leftover Vegetarian Breakfast Burritos	Leftover High-Fiber Mac and Cheese	Farro Risotto *(page 119)*
Day 5	Gingerbread Pancakes *(page 100)*	Leftover Farro Risotto	Santa Fe Cobb Salad *(page 111)*
Day 6	Overnight Steel-Cut Oats *(page 97)*	Leftover Santa Fe Cobb Salad	Jambalaya *(page 108)*
Day 7	Breakfast Ice Cream *(page 95)*	Leftover Jambalaya	Turkey Chili *(page 107)*

Week 2 Shopping List: High-Fiber

CANNED GOODS

Applesauce, unsweetened
Baked beans, in molasses (1 [15-ounce] can)
Black beans (2 [18-ounce] cans)
Chicken stock (1 quart)
Corn, roasted, canned (1)
Kidney beans, no salt added (1 [15-ounce] can)
Lentils, brown or green (3 [15-ounce] cans)
Orange juice
Tomato paste (1 [6-ounce] can)
Tomatoes, crushed (2 [15-ounce] cans)
Tomatoes, diced, no salt added (1 [15-ounce] can)

CONDIMENTS AND SAUCES

Dijon mustard
Hot sauce
Peanut butter
Salad dressing, ranch, blue cheese, or chipotle
Salsa
Vinegar, rice wine

DAIRY AND EGGS

Butter or margarine
Cheddar cheese, sharp, shredded (20 ounces)
Eggs, large
Goat cheese, crumbled (4 ounces)
Greek yogurt, plain
Half-and-half or whipping cream
Milk
Parmesan cheese, grated (4 ounces)
Whipping cream

FREEZER SECTION

Edamame, shelled, frozen
Peas and carrots, mixed, frozen
Raspberries or blackberries, frozen

PRODUCE

Avocados (6)
Bananas (7)
Bell peppers, green (5)
Bell pepper, red or orange (1)
Carrots (3)
Celery (1 head)
English cucumber (1)
Garlic (1 bulb)

Green onions (2 bunches)
Lettuce, romaine (1 large head)
Mushrooms (24 ounces)
Onion, red (1)
Onion, white or Spanish (3)
Orange (1)
Radishes (1 bunch)
Spinach (16 ounces)
Tomatoes (2)
Tomatoes, cherry (12 ounces)
Zucchini (1)

MEAT AND FISH

Bacon
Chicken breast, boneless, skinless (1)
Chicken, ground (½ pound)
Shrimp, large, peeled and deveined (½ pound)
Turkey, lean ground (1 pound)

GRAINS AND STARCHES

Farro
Macaroni, elbow, whole-wheat or high-fiber
Rice, brown basmati
Sesame seeds, black
Tortillas, whole-grain

BAKING AISLE

Almonds, sliced
Baking powder
Baking soda
Chia seeds
Cocoa powder, unsweetened dark
Cranberries, dried unsweetened
Flaxseed, ground
Flour, all-purpose
Flour, whole-wheat
Hemp seeds
Honey
Molasses
Oats, steel-cut
Oil, canola
Oil, olive
Oil, vegetable
Sugar
Vanilla extract

HERBS AND SPICES

- Cajun seasoning
- Chili flakes, crushed red
- Chili powder
- Cinnamon, ground
- Cloves, ground
- Cumin, ground
- Freshly ground black pepper
- Ginger, ground
- Italian seasoning
- Nutmeg, ground
- Onion powder
- Salt

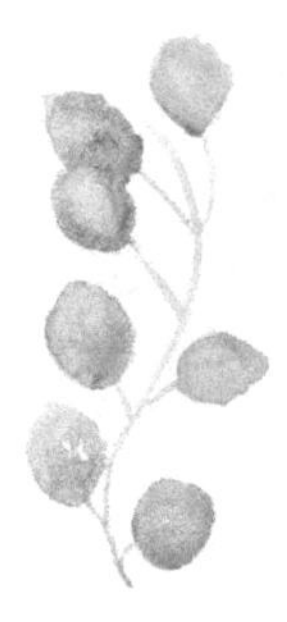

Week 3: High-Fiber

	BREAKFAST	LUNCH	DINNER
Day 1	Breakfast Ice Cream *(page 95)*	Leftover Turkey Chili *(from Week 2)*	Taco Salad *(page 110)*
Day 2	Gingerbread Pancakes *(page 100)*	Leftover Taco Salad	Black Bean Burgers *(page 120)*
Day 3	Overnight Steel-Cut Oats *(page 97)*	Leftover Black Bean Burgers	Lentil and Chicken Shepherd's Pie *(page 122)*
Day 4	High-Fiber Bran Muffins *(page 98)*	Leftover Lentil and Chicken Shepherd's Pie	Jambalaya *(page 108)*
Day 5	Leftover Overnight Steel-Cut Oats	Leftover Jambalaya	Meat Sauce with Lentils *(page 124)*
Day 6	Leftover High-Fiber Bran Muffins	Leftover Meat Sauce with Lentils	Creamy Potato Soup *(page 105)*
Day 7	Quinoa and Avocado Scramble *(page 101)*	Leftover Creamy Potato Soup	Taco Salad *(page 110)*

Week 3 Shopping List: High-Fiber

CANNED GOODS

Applesauce, unsweetened
Black beans (3 [15½-ounce] cans)
Chicken stock (2 quarts)
Kidney beans, white (1 [15½-ounce] can)
Lentils, canned (brown or green) (3 [15-ounce] cans)
Salsa, chunky
Tomatoes, crushed (2 [15-ounce] cans)

CONDIMENTS AND SAUCES

Dijon mustard

DAIRY AND EGGS

Cheddar cheese, shredded (16 ounces)
Eggs, large
Greek yogurt, plain
Milk
Sour cream

FREEZER SECTION

Peas, carrots, and corn, mixed, frozen
Raspberries or blackberries, frozen

PRODUCE

Avocados (2)
Bananas (4)
Bell peppers, green (3)
Bell peppers, red (3)
Berries of your choice (4 ounces)
Celery (1 head)
Cucumber, English (1)
Garlic (1 bulb)
Green onions (3 bunches)
Lettuce, romaine (1 large head)
Lime juice
Mushrooms (32 ounces)
Onions, white or Spanish (3)
Potatoes, russet (8)
Tomatoes, Roma (3)
Zucchini (1)

MEAT AND FISH

Chicken, ground (1 pound)
Chicken breast, boneless, skinless (1)
Shrimp, large, peeled and deveined (½ pound)
Turkey or chicken, lean ground (½ pound)

BAKING AISLE

Baking powder
Baking soda
Chia seeds
Cornstarch
Flour, whole-what
Hemp seeds
Honey or maple syrup
Molasses
Oats, steel-cut
Oil, canola
Oil, vegetable
Sugar
Wheat bran

GRAINS AND STARCHES

Bread crumbs
Burger buns, whole-wheat (4)
Quinoa
Rice, brown basmati

HERBS AND SPICES

Cajun seasoning
Cinnamon, ground
Cloves, ground
Freshly ground black pepper
Garlic powder
Ginger, ground
Italian seasoning
Onion powder
Rosemary, dried
Salt
Taco seasoning
Thyme, dried

Week 4: High-Fiber

	BREAKFAST	LUNCH	DINNER
Day 1	Overnight Steel-Cut Oats *(page 97)*	Leftover Taco Salad *(from Week 3)*	Jambalaya *(page 108)*
Day 2	Quinoa and Avocado Scramble *(page 101)*	Leftover Jambalaya	Lentil and Chicken Shepherd's Pie *(page 122)*
Day 3	Leftover Overnight Steel-Cut Oats	Leftover Lentil and Chicken Shepherd's Pie	Creamy Potato Soup *(page 105)*
Day 4	Breakfast Ice Cream *(page 95)*	Leftover Creamy Potato Soup	Meat Sauce with Lentils *(page 124)*
Day 5	Gingerbread Pancakes *(page 100)*	Leftover Meat Sauce with Lentils	Black Bean Burgers *(page 120)*
Day 6	Leftover Breakfast Ice Cream	Leftover Black Bean Burgers	Taco Salad *(page 110)*
Day 7	High-Fiber Bran Muffins *(page 98)*	Leftover Taco Salad	Leftover Black Bean Burgers

Week 4 Shopping List: High-Fiber

CANNED GOODS

- Applesauce, unsweetened
- Black beans (2 [15½-ounce] cans)
- Chicken stock (2 quarts)
- Kidney beans, white (1 [15½-ounce] can)
- Lentils, canned (brown or green) (3 [15-ounce] cans)
- Salsa, chunky
- Tomatoes, crushed (2 [15-ounce] cans)

CONDIMENTS AND SAUCES

- Dijon mustard

DAIRY AND EGGS

- Cheddar cheese, shredded (16 ounces)
- Eggs, large
- Greek yogurt, plain
- Milk
- Sour cream

FREEZER SECTION

- Peas, carrots, and corn, mixed, frozen
- Raspberries or blackberries, frozen

PRODUCE

- Avocados (2)
- Bananas (4)
- Bell peppers, green (3)
- Bell peppers, red (3)
- Berries of your choice (4 ounces)
- Celery (1 head)
- Cucumber, English (1)
- Garlic (1 bulb)
- Green onions (3 bunches)
- Lettuce, romaine (1 large head)
- Lime juice
- Mushrooms (32 ounces)
- Onions, white or Spanish (3)
- Potatoes, russet (8)
- Tomatoes, Roma (3)
- Zucchini (1)

MEAT AND FISH

- Chicken, ground (1 pound)
- Chicken breast, boneless, skinless (1)
- Shrimp, large, peeled and deveined (½ pound)
- Turkey or chicken, lean, ground (½ pound)

BAKING AISLE

Baking powder
Baking soda
Chia seeds
Cornstarch
Flour, whole-wheat
Hemp seeds
Honey or maple syrup
Molasses
Oats, steel-cut
Oil, canola
Oil, vegetable
Sugar
Wheat bran

GRAINS AND STARCHES

Bread crumbs
Burger buns, whole-wheat (4)
Quinoa
Rice, brown basmati

HERBS AND SPICES

Cajun seasoning
Cinnamon, ground
Cloves, ground
Freshly ground black pepper
Garlic powder
Ginger, ground
Italian seasoning
Onion powder
Rosemary, dried
Salt
Taco seasoning
Thyme, dried

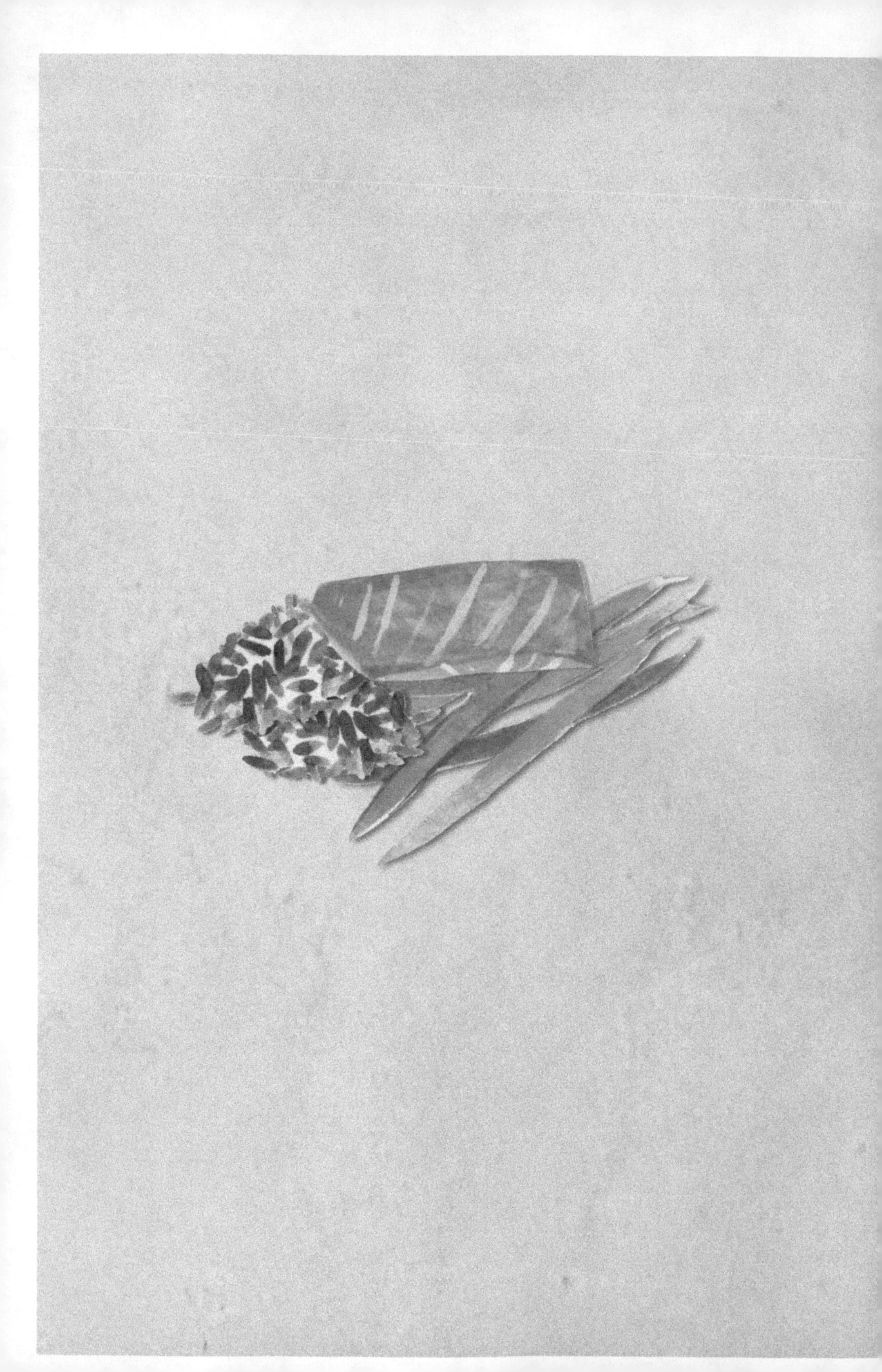

Part II.

The Recipes

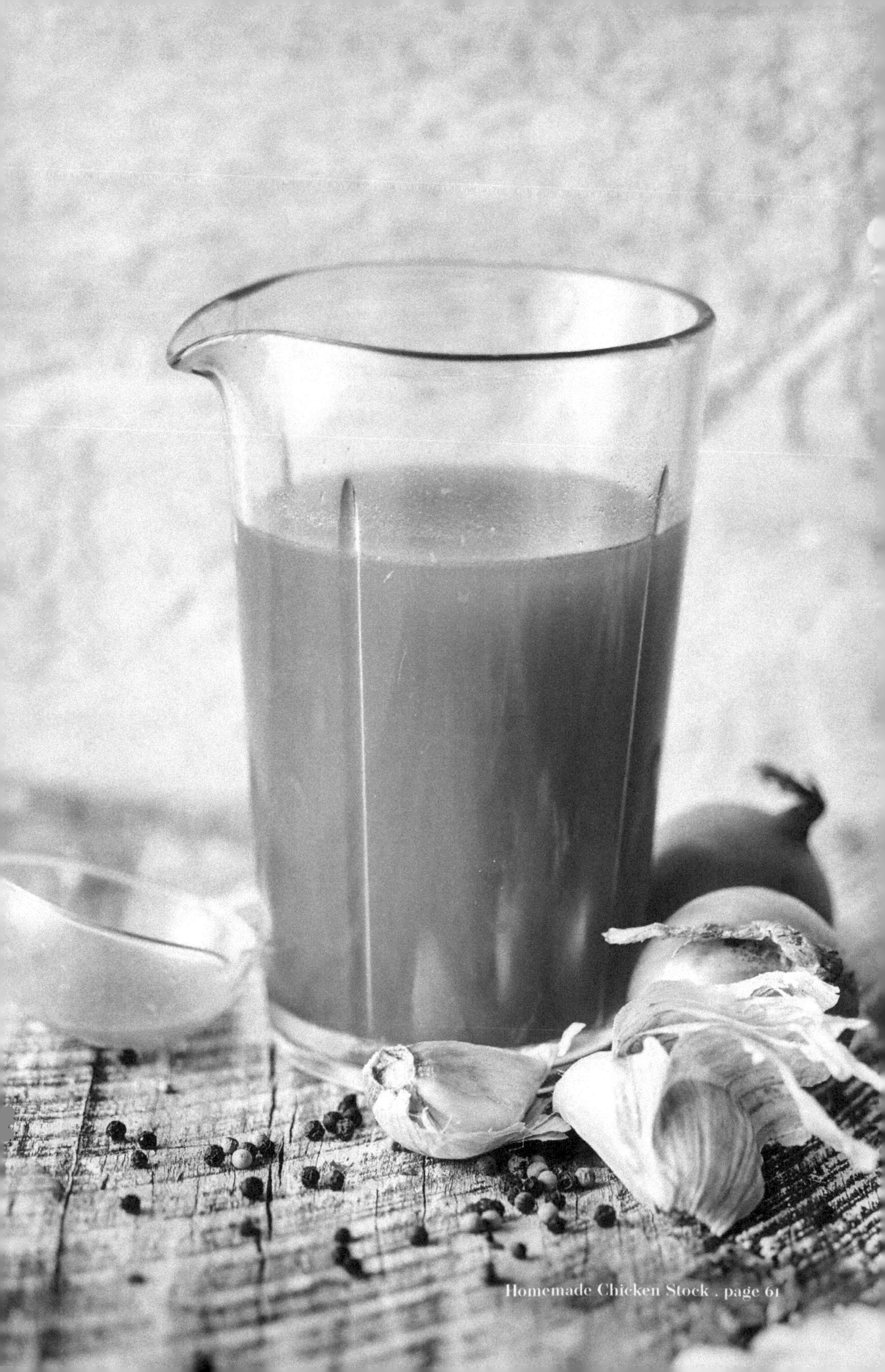
Homemade Chicken Stock . page 61

4.
Clear Fluids

Apple-Cinnamon Tea

Serves 4

Prep time: 5 minutes / Cook time: 25 minutes

With flavors of cinnamon, apple, and a hint of bergamot from the Earl Grey tea, this soothing tea will have you reminiscing about fall days. Plus, it's as pleasing to the nose as it is to the tongue. Fill your home with apple-cinnamon goodness and soothe your body at the same time.

1 cup chopped apples, Honey Crisp, Fuji, Granny Smith, or Gala
3 cinnamon sticks
1 quart water
2 bags Earl Grey tea (caffeinated or decaffeinated)
⅓ cup honey, plus more if desired

1. In a large saucepan over high heat, place the apples, cinnamon sticks, and water and bring to a boil. Lower the heat to medium and simmer for 15 minutes.
2. Remove from the heat and add the Earl Grey tea bags. Steep for 10 minutes.
3. Using a slotted spoon, remove the tea bags, apples, and cinnamon sticks. Add the honey and stir until it dissolves. Taste and add more honey, if desired. Serve hot.
4. Store leftovers in an airtight container in the refrigerator for up to 5 days. Enjoy cold or reheat in the microwave for 1 minute until hot.

Helpful Hint: Make this a ginger cinnamon tea by swapping the apples for ¼ cup minced fresh ginger and the Earl Grey tea for the zest and juice of 1 lemon (juice strained).

Per serving (1 cup): Calories: 101; Fat: <1g; Carbohydrates: 27g; Fiber: 1g; Protein: <1g; Sodium: 6mg; Vitamin B12: 0%; Iron: 1%

Blueberry Green Tea

Serves 4

Cook time: 15 minutes

Did you know that blueberries not only are rich in fiber but are also one of the most nutrient-dense berries? They're packed with vitamin C, vitamin K, and manganese along with antioxidants called flavonoids. This blueberry tea has a hint of tartness balanced by the sweetness of the honey.

½ cup fresh or frozen blueberries

1 quart water

2 bags green tea (caffeinated or decaffeinated)

⅓ cup honey, plus more if desired

clear fluids

1. In a large saucepan over high heat, place the blueberries and water and bring to a boil. Lower the heat to medium and simmer for 5 minutes.
2. Remove from the heat and add the green tea bags. Steep for 10 minutes.
3. Using a slotted spoon, remove the tea bags and blueberries. Add the honey and stir until it dissolves. Taste and add more honey, if desired. Serve hot.
4. Store leftovers in an airtight container in the refrigerator for up to 5 days. Enjoy cold or reheat in the microwave for 1 minute until hot.

Per serving (1 cup): Calories: 95; Fat: 0g; Carbohydrates: 26g; Fiber: 1g; Protein: <1g; Sodium: 7mg; Vitamin B12: 0%; Iron: 1%

Citrus Sports Drink

Serves 8

Prep time: 5 minutes

Some people reach for commercial sports drinks for a quick electrolyte boost, but many store-bought brands don't actually contain electrolytes. To make matters worse, they're typically loaded with sugar or sugar substitutes. With coconut water for natural electrolytes and a bright citrusy flavor, this homemade sports drink is a great way to keep hydrated if you're having trouble with vomiting or diarrhea.

4 cups coconut water
Juice of 4 large oranges (about 1½ cups), strained
2 tablespoons lemon juice, strained
2 tablespoons honey or maple syrup
1 teaspoon sea salt

1. Place the coconut water, orange juice, lemon juice, honey, and salt in a jug or pitcher and stir until the salt is dissolved. Serve cold.
2. Store in the refrigerator for up to 5 days.

Per serving (1 cup): Calories: 59; Fat: <1g; Carbohydrates: 14g; Fiber: <1g; Protein: <1g; Sodium: 304mg; Vitamin B12: 0%; Iron: 1%

Homemade Orange Gelatin

Serves 4

Prep time: 10 minutes, plus 4 hours chilling time / Cook time: 3 minutes

Most Americans are no stranger to flavored gelatin, but have you made it from scratch before? This homemade gelatin is healthier for you than the instant version, with all-natural ingredients, a tangy orange flavor, and no artificial sweeteners. It's not much harder to make than the packaged version, either.

Juice of 8 large oranges (about 3 cups), strained and divided

2 tablespoons unflavored gelatin

2 tablespoons honey or maple syrup

1. In a large bowl, pour in ½ cup of orange juice and sprinkle with gelatin. Whisk well and let sit for 5 minutes, until the gelatin begins to set but is not quite smooth.
2. In a medium saucepan over low heat, pour in the remaining 2½ cups of orange juice and cook until just before boiling, 2 to 3 minutes.
3. Remove from the heat and pour the hot juice into the gelatin mixture. Add the honey or maple syrup and stir until the gelatin is dissolved.
4. Pour into an 8-by-8-inch baking dish and transfer to the refrigerator. Refrigerate for 4 hours to set. Serve cold.
5. To store, cover the dish with plastic wrap and refrigerate for up to 5 days.

Helpful Hint: Swap the fruit juice in this gelatin for a number of different flavors. I recommend lemon, lime, or even peach. Just be sure your fruit juice is pulp-free.

Per serving (1 4-inch square): Calories: 127; Fat: <1g; Carbohydrates: 28g; Fiber: <1g; Protein: 6g; Sodium: 2mg; Vitamin B12: 0%; Iron: 2%

Raspberry Lemonade Ice Pops

Makes 4 ice pops

Prep time: 10 minutes, plus 4 hours chilling time

When you're on a clear fluid diet, it's easy to get tired of the lack of texture. Soup and tea are soothing, but these ice pops provide a much-needed crunch that tastes just like raspberry lemonade. They're made with coconut water, a natural electrolyte that will help rehydrate you after you've been sick.

3 cups frozen raspberries

1 teaspoon lemon juice, strained

¼ cup coconut water

¼ cup honey or maple syrup

1. In a blender, puree the raspberries, lemon juice, and coconut water until smooth.
2. Pour the mixture through a fine mesh strainer into a bowl to remove the seeds. Stir in the honey until well mixed.
3. Divide the mixture equally among 4 popsicle molds and freeze until solid, 3 to 4 hours.

Helpful Hint: You may want to stock up on ice pop molds during warmer months, as they can be hard to find in the winter.

Per serving (1 ice pop): Calories: 120; Fat: 0g; Carbohydrates: 31g; Fiber: 7g; Protein: 2g; Sodium: 2mg; Vitamin B12: 0%; Iron: 1%

Tropical Ice Pops

Makes 4 ice pops

Prep time: 10 minutes, plus 4 hours chilling time

Ice pops are delicious any time of year, but these tropical pops are especially delicious when it's warm. If you're feeling nauseated, they will help rehydrate your body and even give you a little boost of energy.

Juice of 8 oranges (about 3 cups), strained

¼ cup coconut water

1 teaspoon lemon juice, strained

¼ cup honey or maple syrup

1. In a bowl, mix together the orange juice, coconut water, and lemon juice.
2. Pour the mixture through a fine mesh strainer into a bowl to remove any seeds.
3. Stir in the honey until well mixed.
4. Pour the mixture into popsicle molds and freeze until solid, 3 to 4 hours.

Helpful Hint: You may want to stock up on ice pop molds during warmer months, as they can be hard to find in the winter.

Per serving (1 ice pop): Calories: 151; Fat: <1g; Carbohydrates: 37g; Fiber: <1g; Protein: 1g; Sodium: 4mg; Vitamin B12: 0%; Iron: 3%

Homemade Beef Stock

Serves 6

Prep time: 10 minutes / Cook time: 2½ to 12½ hours

This beef stock is rich in both flavor and nutrients. It's a great recipe to freeze in smaller containers and use later as a base for gravies, roasts, and soups once you're off the clear fluid diet.

- **2 pounds beef bones (preferably with marrow)**
- **5 celery stalks, chopped**
- **4 carrots, chopped**
- **1 white or Spanish onion, chopped**
- **2 garlic cloves, crushed**
- **2 bay leaves**
- **1 teaspoon dried thyme**
- **1 teaspoon dried sage**
- **1 teaspoon black peppercorns**
- **Salt**

1. Preheat the oven to 425°F.
2. On a large baking sheet, spread out the beef bones, celery, carrots, onion, garlic, and bay leaves. Sprinkle the thyme, sage, and peppercorns over the top.
3. Roast for 20 to 30 minutes, or until the vegetables and bones have a rich brown color.
4. Transfer the roasted bones and vegetables to a large stockpot. Cover with water and slowly bring to a boil over high heat. Lower the heat to medium-low and simmer for at least 2 hours and up to 12 hours. (The longer it cooks, the more flavor you will get.)
5. Carefully pour the mixture through a fine mesh strainer into a large bowl. Taste and season with salt. Serve hot.
6. Store in airtight containers in the refrigerator for up to 5 days or in the freezer for up to 4 months.

Helpful Hint: You can also make this stock in a slow cooker set on high. I typically start cooking my stock in the late evening, and I strain it when I wake up the next morning.

Per serving: Calories: 37; Fat: 1g; Carbohydrates: 3g; Fiber: 0g; Protein: 4g; Sodium: 58mg; Vitamin B12: 0%; Iron: 0%

Homemade Chicken Stock

Serves 6

Prep time: 10 minutes / Cook time: 2½ to 12½ hours

While you're on a clear fluid diet, this stock is the next best thing to the comfort of chicken soup. And later on, you can use it in any recipe that calls for chicken stock. Your body will thank you for this healing broth that's much lower in salt than store-bought versions.

1 (2-pound) chicken carcass
5 celery stalks, chopped
4 carrots, chopped
1 white or Spanish onion, chopped
2 garlic cloves, crushed
2 bay leaves
1 teaspoon dried thyme
1 teaspoon dried sage
1 teaspoon black peppercorns
Salt

1. Preheat the oven to 425°F.
2. On a large baking sheet, spread out the chicken bones, celery, carrots, onion, garlic, and bay leaves. Sprinkle the thyme, sage, and peppercorns over the top. Roast for 20 to 30 minutes, or until the vegetables and bones have a rich brown color.
3. Transfer the roasted bones and vegetables to a large stockpot. Add 6 quarts of water and slowly bring to a boil over high heat. Lower the heat to medium-low and simmer for at least 2 hours and up to 12 hours. (The longer it cooks, the more flavor you will get.)
4. Carefully pour the mixture through a fine mesh strainer into a large bowl. Season with salt and serve hot.
5. Store in airtight containers in the refrigerator for up to 5 days or in the freezer for up to 4 months.

Helpful Hint: Feel free to combine all the ingredients in a slow cooker instead. Before you go to bed, set it on high, and strain the stock the next morning.

Per serving: Calories: 33; Fat: 1g; Carbohydrates: 3g; Fiber: 0g; Protein: 3g; Sodium: 20mg; Vitamin B12: 0%; Iron: 0%

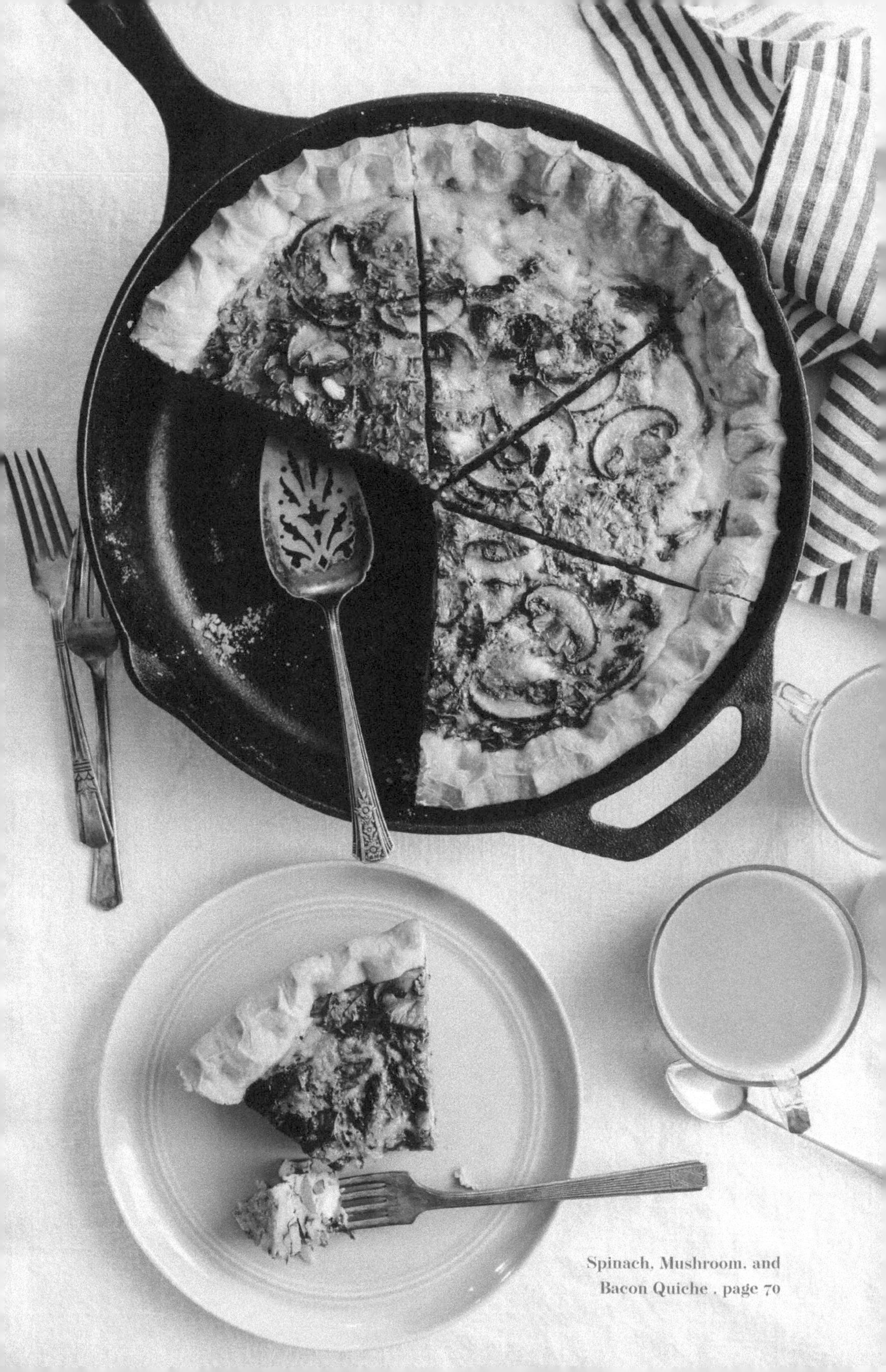

Spinach, Mushroom, and
Bacon Quiche . page 70

5.

Low-Residue Recipes

Strawberry Cheesecake Smoothie

Serves 2

Prep time: 5 minutes

For a smoothie that tastes exactly like cheesecake, it's surprisingly healthy. The cottage cheese gives it a protein kick, and the strawberries bring a nice tartness. Make this smoothie as an on-the-go breakfast—with just five ingredients, it's done practically in seconds, and you're out the door!

2 cups frozen strawberries
1 cup milk
1 cup cottage cheese
3 tablespoons honey or maple syrup
1 teaspoon vanilla extract

In a blender or food processor, puree the strawberries, milk, cottage cheese, honey, and vanilla until smooth. Serve immediately.

Helpful Hint: If you or your family are dairy-free, you can substitute almond milk, rice milk, coconut milk, soy milk, or oat milk for the dairy milk. Whichever nondairy milk you choose, be sure it is calcium-fortified so you're not missing out on any nutrients.

Per serving: Calories: 297; Fat: 4g; Carbohydrates: 50g; Fiber: 3g; Protein: 18g; Sodium: 431mg; Vitamin B12: 22%; Iron: 8%

Apple-Cinnamon Muffins

Makes 12 muffins

Prep time: 15 minutes / Cook time: 25 minutes

These muffins make the perfect complement to a bowl of high-protein Greek yogurt, a handful of nuts, or a piece of cheese, making a complete, healthy breakfast. Pop one in your bag when you're traveling or out and about for a snack between meals.

2 cups all-purpose flour

½ cup sugar

2 teaspoons ground cinnamon

1 teaspoon baking powder

½ teaspoon baking soda

¾ cup unsweetened applesauce

2 apples, Honey Crisp, Fuji, Granny Smith, or Gala, peeled and grated

1 teaspoon vanilla extract

1 large egg

4 tablespoons (½ stick) butter or margarine, at room temperature

1. Preheat the oven to 350°F. Line a 12-cup muffin tin with muffin liners and set aside.
2. In a large mixing bowl, mix together the flour, sugar, cinnamon, baking powder, and baking soda.
3. Make a well in the middle of the flour mixture, add the applesauce, grated apples, vanilla, egg, and butter to the well, and gently whisk to combine. Be careful not to overmix, or the muffins will be tough.
4. Spoon the batter equally into the lined muffin cups. Bake for 20 to 25 minutes, or until a toothpick inserted into the center of a muffin comes out clean. Serve warm or at room temperature.
5. Store the muffins in an airtight container at room temperature for up to 5 days.

Per serving (1 muffin): Calories: 160; Fat: 4g; Carbohydrates: 25g; Fiber: 1g; Protein: 3g; Sodium: 127mg; Vitamin B12: 1%; Iron: 6%

Peach Scones

Makes 12 scones

Prep time: 15 minutes / Cook time: 20 minutes

Scones are a great grab-and-go breakfast. This version has its natural sweetness (and vitamin C) from peaches.

- **2½ cups all-purpose flour**
- **½ cup sugar, plus more for sprinkling**
- **1 tablespoon baking powder**
- **1 teaspoon ground cinnamon**
- **½ teaspoon baking soda**
- **¾ teaspoon salt**
- **8 tablespoons (1 stick) cold butter, cut into cubes**
- **1 cup canned peaches packed in water, drained and finely diced**
- **¾ cup milk, plus more for brushing**
- **1 tablespoon vanilla extract**

1. Preheat the oven to 425°F. Line a baking sheet with parchment paper.
2. In a large mixing bowl, mix together the flour, sugar, baking powder, cinnamon, baking soda, and salt.
3. Add the butter and work it into the dry ingredients with a fork or pastry blender until it resembles pea-sized clumps.
4. Add the peaches, milk, and vanilla and mix until a stiff dough forms.
5. Cut the dough in half and form each portion into a disk about 1 inch thick. Run a large knife under cold water and cut each disk into 6 wedges. Transfer the wedges to the prepared baking sheet, brush them with milk, and sprinkle them lightly with sugar.
6. Bake for 15 to 20 minutes, or until the tops are golden. Let cool on a wire rack for 5 minutes before serving.

Per serving (1 scone): Calories: 199; Fat: 8g; Carbohydrates: 29g; Fiber: 1g; Protein: 3g; Sodium: 382mg; Vitamin B12: 1%; Iron: 7%

Classic French Toast

Serves 4

Prep time: 5 minutes / Cook time: 40 minutes

The classic reinvention of day-old bread, French toast is a wonderful way to start your weekend mornings. You might not think of it as a protein-rich dish, but the milk and eggs play a big role in giving this recipe fortitude. Pair it with some seasonal fruit for a complete meal.

1 teaspoon butter or margarine

3 large eggs

½ cup milk

2 teaspoons vanilla extract

2 teaspoons ground cinnamon

8 thick slices day-old white bread of your choice

¼ cup confectioners' sugar or maple syrup, for serving

1. In a large sauté pan or skillet over medium heat, melt the butter.
2. In a medium bowl, whisk together the eggs, milk, vanilla, and cinnamon until smooth.
3. Pour the egg mixture into a large, shallow dish.
4. Dip a slice of bread into the batter, let it soak for 10 to 15 seconds on each side, and immediately place it in the hot skillet. Cook until both sides are golden brown, 2 to 3 minutes per side. Repeat with the remaining slices of bread. Depending on the size of your skillet, you can likely cook 2 slices at once.
5. Place 2 slices of French toast on each plate and dust each serving with 1 tablespoon of confectioners' sugar or lightly drizzle with 1 tablespoon of maple syrup.

Per serving (2 slices): Calories: 353; Fat: 8g; Carbohydrates: 55g; Fiber: 2g; Protein: 12g; Sodium: 374mg; Vitamin B12: 8%; Iron: 22%

Greek Yogurt Banana Pancakes

Serves 4

Prep time: 10 minutes / Cook time: 40 minutes

Thanks to the Greek yogurt, these pancakes are a great way to get your protein in the morning and still satisfy that carb craving. Bananas are a classic pancake pairing, but they play a special role here in keeping the pancakes moist and delicious. Top these with fresh fruit or a dollop of Greek yogurt.

1 teaspoon butter or margarine

1½ cups all-purpose flour

2 tablespoons sugar

1 teaspoon ground cinnamon

1 teaspoon baking powder

½ teaspoon baking soda

Pinch salt

1 banana, mashed

2 large eggs

⅔ cup milk

½ cup plain Greek yogurt

¼ cup maple syrup, for serving

1. In a large sauté pan or skillet over medium heat, melt the butter or margarine.
2. In a large mixing bowl, whisk together the flour, sugar, cinnamon, baking powder, baking soda, and salt.
3. Add the banana, eggs, milk, and Greek yogurt and whisk until just combined. The batter should be thick and slightly lumpy.
4. Pour ¼ cup of batter per pancake into the hot skillet. Cook until bubbles form along the edges, 2 to 3 minutes per side. Repeat with the rest of the batter.
5. Place 2 pancakes on each plate and top with 1 tablespoon of maple syrup per serving.

Per serving (2 pancakes): Calories: 345; Fat: 5g; Carbohydrates: 64g; Fiber: 3g; Protein: 12g; Sodium: 372mg; Vitamin B12: 7%; Iron: 15%

Avocado Eggs

Serves 4

Prep time: 5 minutes / Cook time: 20 minutes

This is a fancy yet easy way to cook an egg that doesn't even require a skillet. Impress your family or friends with this unique, tasty breakfast option and pair it with a slice of white toast. Sometimes the most delicious meals are the simplest.

2 ripe avocados, cut in half and pits removed

4 large eggs

Salt

Freshly ground black pepper

1 cup shredded Cheddar cheese

2 green onions, minced

1. Preheat the oven to 425°F.
2. Place the avocados cut-side up on a baking sheet.
3. Crack 1 egg into each avocado half.
4. Season with salt and pepper and top with the cheese and green onions.
5. Bake for 15 to 20 minutes, until the eggs are cooked to your preference. Serve warm.

Per serving (½ avocado): Calories: 329; Fat: 27g; Carbohydrates: 9g; Fiber: 6g; Protein: 14g; Sodium: 259mg; Vitamin B12: 8%; Iron: 8%

Spinach, Mushroom, and Bacon Quiche

Serves 4

Prep time: 10 minutes / Cook time: 55 minutes

This recipe is a spin on the most well-known quiche dish, quiche florentine, which has spinach, bacon lardons, and cheese. If you want to pack this quiche with even more veggies, add cooked asparagus tips and finely chopped carrots. Quiche is delicious either hot or cold, but I prefer mine hot with a salad on the side.

1 (9-inch) premade pie shell

3 large eggs

1½ cups milk of choice

Pinch salt

Pinch freshly ground black pepper

4 slices bacon or ½ cup precooked bacon bits

1 cup shredded cheese of choice, divided

1 (10-ounce) package frozen spinach, thawed and squeezed dry

½ cup sliced mushrooms

1. Preheat the oven to 375°F.
2. Parbake the pie shell for 5 to 7 minutes. This will prevent the crust from getting soggy after you add the egg mixture. Set aside.
3. In a medium bowl, whisk together the eggs, milk, salt, and pepper. Set aside.
4. Line a plate with paper towels. In a large sauté pan or skillet over medium heat, cook the bacon until crisp, 5 to 7 minutes. Transfer the bacon to the lined plate. When cool, crumble into bits.
5. Sprinkle the pie shell with ½ cup of the cheese. Add the spinach, mushrooms, and bacon.
6. Pour the egg mixture into the pie shell (it should be about ⅔ full). Sprinkle the remaining ½ cup of cheese over the top of the egg mixture.

7. Bake for 30 to 40 minutes, or until the pastry is golden and the egg mixture is just set but still wobbly. Cut into wedges and serve warm, or refrigerate for 1 hour and serve cold.

8. To store, cover the pan with plastic wrap and refrigerate for up to 5 days.

Helpful Hint: This quiche recipe works great for meal prepping. Double the recipe and make 2 quiches. Eat one now and freeze the other one for up to 4 months.

Per serving: Calories: 503; Fat: 31g; Carbohydrates: 35g; Fiber: 2g; Protein: 22g; Sodium: 722mg; Vitamin B12: 15%; Iron: 9%

Creamy Mushroom Soup

Serves 6

Prep time: 10 minutes / Cook time: 35 minutes

This homemade mushroom soup is easy to make and packed with wholesome ingredients. Rich, creamy, and perfect for recovery, this soup is on your table in just 40 minutes.

4 tablespoons (½ stick) butter

1 large white or Spanish onion, diced

1½ pounds button mushrooms, sliced

2 portabella mushrooms, sliced

½ cup pinot grigio or sauvignon blanc wine

6 tablespoons all-purpose flour

2 teaspoons garlic powder

2 teaspoons dried thyme

3 cups vegetable broth

2 cups whipping cream

Salt

Freshly ground black pepper

1. In a large saucepan over medium heat, melt the butter. Add the onion and cook, stirring occasionally, until the onion is fragrant and translucent, 4 to 5 minutes.
2. Add the button and portabella mushrooms and cook until they begin to soften, 2 to 3 minutes. Add the wine and cook, stirring occasionally, for another 2 to 3 minutes.
3. Add the flour, garlic powder, and thyme and stir to combine. Slowly whisk in the vegetable broth and continue to cook until the sauce begins to thicken, about 7 minutes.
4. Slowly whisk in the whipping cream and bring to a boil, about 2 minutes. Lower the heat to low and simmer until heated through, about 15 minutes. Taste, season with salt and pepper, and serve.
5. Store leftovers in an airtight container and refrigerate for up to 5 days.

Per serving: Calories: 434; Fat: 38g; Carbohydrates: 18g; Fiber: 3g; Protein: 7g; Sodium: 563mg; Vitamin B12: 4%; Iron: 11%

Chicken and Rice Soup

Serves 6

Prep time: 10 minutes / Cook time: 30 minutes

When you're recovering from a flare-up, there's nothing more comforting than warm chicken soup. I often save leftover turkey or chicken breast to make this recipe even quicker, and I usually freeze an extra batch for when my family is under the weather. It's like a warm hug in a bowl.

2 tablespoons vegetable oil, divided

¼ cup diced white or Spanish onion

1 bay leaf

½ teaspoon salt

½ teaspoon freshly ground black pepper

1½ cups chopped celery

1½ cups chopped carrots

1 garlic clove, minced

1½ cups diced chicken or turkey breast

3 quarts plus 1 cup Homemade Chicken Stock (page 61) or store-bought chicken stock

1 cup jasmine rice, rinsed

1. In a large stockpot over medium heat, warm 1 tablespoon of oil. Add the onion, bay leaf, salt, and pepper and sauté until the onions are fragrant and translucent, 2 to 3 minutes. Add the celery, carrots, and garlic and cook until the vegetables begin to soften, 2 to 3 minutes.
2. In a large sauté pan or skillet over medium-high heat, warm the remaining 1 tablespoon of oil until it just begins to shimmer. Add the chicken and cook, stirring occasionally, until the chicken has browned, 5 to 7 minutes. The poultry will not be cooked all the way through.
3. Add the chicken and the chicken stock to the stockpot with the vegetables, raise the heat to medium-high, and bring to a boil. Lower the heat to medium, add the rice, and simmer until the rice and vegetables are tender and the poultry has finished cooking, about 12 minutes.

continued ▸

Chicken and Rice Soup continued

4. Remove the bay leaf and ladle the soup into bowls.
5. Leftovers can be stored in an airtight container and refrigerated for up to 5 days or frozen for up to 4 months.

Helpful Hint: If you'd like to amp up the flavor even more, add a pinch each of thyme, basil, and oregano to the simmering stock, or add 2 tablespoons curry powder to the onion mixture in step 1 and ¼ cup coconut milk along with the stock in step 3.

Per serving: Calories: 276; Fat: 9g; Carbohydrates: 34g; Fiber: 2g; Protein: 16g; Sodium: 300mg; Vitamin B12: 0%; Iron: 3%

One-Pot Chicken and Orzo

Serves 6

Prep time: 10 minutes / Cook time: 20 minutes

Orzo may look like rice, but it's actually a form of short-cut pasta with a quick cooking time. This recipe will have dinner on the table in 30 minutes and fewer dishes to clean up because it's a one-pot meal.

1 tablespoon canola oil

1 cup diced chicken breast

1½ cups orzo pasta

4 cups Homemade Chicken Stock (page 61) or store-bought chicken stock

½ cup chopped fresh or frozen and thawed asparagus tips

½ teaspoon garlic powder

1 teaspoon onion powder

1½ cups frozen mixed peas and carrots

Salt

Freshly ground black pepper

½ cup grated Parmesan cheese

1. In a large sauté pan or skillet over medium heat, warm the oil until it just begins to shimmer. Add the chicken and cook, stirring occasionally, until it's browned but not yet cooked through, about 5 minutes. Add the orzo and cook until the pasta has slightly softened, about 1 minute.
2. Raise the heat to medium-high, add the chicken stock, asparagus tips, garlic powder, and onion powder, and bring to a boil. Lower the heat to medium-low and simmer until the asparagus is tender and the chicken is cooked through, 8 to 10 minutes.
3. Stir in the frozen peas and carrots and cook until heated through, about 2 minutes.
4. Taste and season with salt and pepper. Sprinkle with the Parmesan cheese. Serve hot.

Helpful Hint: Use leftover cooked chicken breast to make this 30-minute meal even quicker.

Per serving: Calories: 306; Fat: 8g; Carbohydrates: 38g; Fiber: 3g; Protein: 19g; Sodium: 211mg; Vitamin B12: 2%; Iron: 12%

Shrimp Curry

Serves 4

Prep time: 10 minutes / Cook time: 35 minutes

Shrimp curry is a common dish in Thai cuisine. This rich curry dish is packed with flavor and amazing aromas. Serve it over steamed white rice to complete this meal. This is a quick curry, which makes it perfect for busy weekday nights.

1½ cups jasmine rice, rinsed

2¼ cups water

¼ teaspoon vegetable oil

1 pound large shrimp, peeled and deveined

Salt

Freshly ground black pepper

2 tablespoons butter or margarine

1 white or Spanish onion, diced

1 garlic clove, minced

1 (6-ounce) can tomato paste

1 tablespoon yellow curry paste

½ teaspoon ground ginger

1 tablespoon all-purpose flour

1 (13½-ounce) can unsweetened coconut milk

1 teaspoon lime juice

1 teaspoon honey

¼ cup chopped fresh cilantro (optional)

1. In a medium saucepan over high heat, mix the rice with 2¼ cups water and bring to a boil. Lower the heat to medium-low, cover, and cook for 10 minutes. Remove from the heat and let sit, covered, for an additional 10 minutes.
2. In a large sauté pan or skillet over medium heat, warm the oil until it just begins to shimmer. Add the shrimp and season with salt and pepper. Cook, stirring occasionally, until the shrimp are bright pink, 3 to 5 minutes. Remove the shrimp from the pan and set aside.
3. Add the butter and onion to the pan and cook until the onion is fragrant and translucent, 3 to 4 minutes. Add the garlic, tomato paste, curry paste, and ginger and stir to combine. Add the flour and cook, stirring, for 1 to 2 minutes.
4. Slowly whisk in the coconut milk until the sauce is smooth. Simmer until it begins to thicken, 5 to 7 minutes.

5. Add the lime juice and honey and stir. Return the shrimp to the pan and stir to combine. Taste and season with salt and pepper, if needed.
6. Serve warm over the steamed rice. Garnish with the cilantro, if using.

Per serving: Calories: 647; Fat: 27g; Carbohydrates: 69g; Fiber: 3g; Protein: 32g; Sodium: 760mg; Vitamin B12: 22%; Iron: 26%

Pad Thai

Serves 4

Prep time: 10 minutes / Cook time: 15 minutes

Pad Thai is traditional street food in parts of Thailand, so it probably shouldn't come as a surprise that it's easy to make at home. Customize this dish however you like: Swap out the shrimp for chicken breast or thigh, or add in a scrambled egg.

10 ounces flat rice noodles

¼ cup tamarind paste

2 tablespoons soy sauce

2 tablespoons rice vinegar

2 tablespoons fish sauce

¼ teaspoon sriracha sauce

1 garlic clove, minced

1 tablespoon water

2 teaspoons peanut oil

1 pound large shrimp, peeled and deveined

2 carrots, julienned

1 cup bean sprouts

1 red bell pepper, finely diced

4 green onions, minced

½ cup chopped fresh cilantro (optional)

1 lime, cut into 8 wedges

1. In a medium bowl, cover the rice noodles in cold water, soak for 5 minutes, and drain.
2. In a small bowl, mix together the tamarind paste, soy sauce, rice vinegar, fish sauce, sriracha, garlic, and water. Set aside.
3. In a large sauté pan or skillet over medium heat, warm the peanut oil until it begins to shimmer. Add the shrimp, carrots, and bean sprouts and cook, stirring occasionally, until the shrimp begin to turn pink and the vegetables have started to soften, about 5 minutes. Add the bell pepper and green onions, stir, and cook until the shrimp are cooked through and the peppers are tender, 4 to 5 more minutes.

4. Add the rice noodles and sauce to the pan and mix until the noodles are well coated.
5. Garnish with chopped cilantro (if using) and a squeeze of fresh lime juice. Serve immediately.

Helpful Hint: If you don't have tamarind paste, you can substitute a mixture of 1 tablespoon brown sugar and 2 tablespoons lime juice.

Per serving: Calories: 504; Fat: 6g; Carbohydrates: 84g; Fiber: 6g; Protein: 31g; Sodium: 1,493mg; Vitamin B12: 23%; Iron: 28%

Salmon Cakes

Serves 6

Prep time: 10 minutes / Cook time: 20 minutes

Salmon is an amazing lean protein that's packed with omega-3 fatty acids. This preparation is similar to crab cakes, except you can eat these cakes on a bun. I like to make them for backyard barbecues, but they're great anytime you want a unique, delicious meal.

½ pound salmon, bones and skin removed, diced
2 garlic cloves, minced
1 large egg
¾ cup bread crumbs
¼ cup minced chives
1 tablespoon lemon juice
1 teaspoon hot sauce
½ teaspoon Dijon mustard
½ teaspoon salt
½ teaspoon freshly ground black pepper
¼ teaspoon paprika
1 tablespoon vegetable oil
6 white burger buns, toasted

1. In a large bowl, mix together the salmon, garlic, egg, bread crumbs, chives, lemon juice, hot sauce, Dijon mustard, salt, pepper, and paprika until just combined.
2. Form the mixture into 6 patties.
3. In a large sauté pan or skillet over medium heat, warm the oil until it begins to shimmer. Add the salmon patties and cook until the salmon begins to turn pink and the bottom is browned, 7 to 10 minutes. Flip and cook until the patties are firm and golden on both sides, another 7 to 10 minutes. The salmon should be pale pink.
4. Serve the patties hot, sandwiched between the toasted buns.
5. Leftover salmon cakes can be stored in an airtight container in the refrigerator for up to 5 days or in the freezer for up to 3 months.

Helpful Hint: Try spreading some spicy mayo on the bun for a pop of extra flavor.

Per serving (1 cake): Calories: 225; Fat: 6g; Carbohydrates: 29g; Fiber: 1g; Protein: 13g; Sodium: 456mg; Vitamin B12: 1%; Iron: 10%

Cod en Papillote

Serves 4

Prep time: 15 minutes / Cook time: 25 minutes

En papillote *is French for "in paper"—parchment paper, in this case. When you use this method, the cod and veggies bake inside a folded pouch that traps steam, keeping everything moist as it cooks.*

2 Yukon Gold potatoes, very thinly sliced

1 cup chopped asparagus tips

1 red bell pepper, thinly sliced

¼ red onion, very thinly sliced

4 teaspoons butter

Salt

Freshly ground black pepper

4 (5-ounce) cod fillets, bones and skin removed

4 very thin lemon slices

1. Preheat the oven to 400°F. Cut 4 (12-inch) sheets of parchment paper and fold them each in half. Open them up and turn them so the fold is horizontal on the counter in front of you.
2. Place ¼ of the potatoes on the bottom half of each piece of parchment. Repeat this process with ¼ of the asparagus, bell pepper, red onion, and butter. Season each portion with salt and pepper.
3. Place 1 cod fillet on top of each pile of vegetables and sprinkle with more salt and pepper. Place 1 slice of lemon on each piece of fish.
4. To seal the packages, fold the top half of the parchment paper over the vegetables and fish. Starting at one corner, fold the edges over, pinching as you go, until the packet is closed. Repeat with the remaining pouches.
5. Bake for 20 to 25 minutes, until the fish is cooked through and the vegetables are tender. Serve hot in the packet, carefully opening the paper to avoid the escaping steam.

Per serving: Calories: 262; Fat: 5g; Carbohydrates: 20g; Fiber: 4g; Protein: 35g; Sodium: 140mg; Vitamin B12: 25%; Iron: 10%

Panzanella Salad

Serves 4

Prep time: 10 minutes / Cook time: 10 minutes

Panzanella is a traditional Italian bread salad from the region of Tuscany. It's a great way to use up dry, day-old white bread or croutons. This salad is full of juicy tomatoes, fresh basil, and cucumbers for lots of crunch. Plus, the bocconcini (little balls of mozzarella) give it a luscious richness. It is an ideal make-ahead salad because it can sit for up to 8 hours in the refrigerator.

Day-old or stale French bread, cut into large cubes

¼ cup olive oil

2 tablespoons balsamic vinegar

1 teaspoon honey

4 Roma tomatoes, cut into large dice

¼ peeled English cucumber, cut into large dice

½ cup bocconcini

¼ cup chopped fresh basil

Salt

Freshly ground black pepper

1. Preheat the oven to 375°F. Line a baking sheet with parchment paper.
2. Place the cubed bread on the prepared baking sheet and bake for 10 minutes, or until golden brown. Let cool.
3. In a small bowl, mix together the oil, balsamic vinegar, and honey.
4. In a large bowl, toss together the tomatoes, cucumber, bocconcini, bread, and basil until combined.
5. Drizzle the dressing lightly over the salad and toss to combine.
6. Taste and season with salt and pepper, if needed.

Per serving: Calories: 479; Fat: 21g; Carbohydrates: 62g; Fiber: 4g; Protein: 13g; Sodium: 622mg; Vitamin B12: 0%; Iron: 18%

Stuffed Mushrooms

Serves 4

Prep time: 15 minutes / Cook time: 25 minutes

Because of their high water content, mushrooms are a great choice to help manage your symptoms. And they are the only vegetable that naturally contains vitamin D. How great is that? These stuffed mushrooms make a great addition to any meal or potluck.

4 portabella mushrooms (about 1 pound)
Salt
Freshly ground black pepper
1 tablespoon olive oil
1 cup finely chopped baby spinach
¼ cup finely chopped green onion
1 garlic clove, minced
½ cup bread crumbs
¼ cup grated Parmesan cheese

1. Preheat the oven to 350°F. Grease a 9-by-13-inch baking dish.
2. Clean the mushrooms with a damp paper towel. Remove the stems and set the caps aside. Finely chop the stems and set aside.
3. Place the caps upside down in the prepared baking dish. Lightly season with salt and pepper.
4. In a large sauté pan or skillet over medium heat, warm the oil. Add the spinach, onion, and garlic and cook until the vegetables are tender, 4 to 5 minutes.
5. Remove from heat and stir in the bread crumbs. Season lightly with salt and pepper.
6. Spoon the mixture into the mushroom caps and top with the Parmesan cheese.
7. Bake for 15 to 20 minutes, or until the mushrooms are tender.

Per serving: Calories: 135; Fat: 6g; Carbohydrates: 16g; Fiber: 3g; Protein: 7g; Sodium: 154mg; Vitamin B12: 2%; Iron: 7%

Balsamic Roasted Carrots

Serves 6

Prep time: 10 minutes / Cook time: 40 minutes

Carrots are a low-fiber vegetable that's great for managing diverticulitis, but they also have other health benefits. The beta carotene and antioxidants in carrots have been linked to reducing the risk of cancer, lowering cholesterol levels, and improving eye health.

2 tablespoons maple syrup

2 tablespoons balsamic vinegar

1 tablespoon canola oil or grape seed oil

½ teaspoon garlic powder

¼ teaspoon ground ginger

Pinch salt

Pinch freshly ground black pepper

10 medium carrots peeled and cut in half lengthwise (or in quarters if they are large)

1. Preheat the oven to 400°F. Line a baking sheet with parchment paper or aluminum foil.
2. In a small bowl, mix together the maple syrup, balsamic vinegar, oil, garlic powder, ginger, salt, and pepper.
3. Place the carrots on the prepared baking sheet and drizzle with half of the maple syrup mixture. Toss the carrots until they are coated in the glaze. Roast for 15 to 20 minutes, or until the carrots start to caramelize.
4. Flip the carrots, pour the remaining half of the glaze over the top, and roast for another 15 to 20 minutes, until the carrots are tender and cooked through.

Helpful Hint: I really like the beautiful restaurant-style carrots at Costco that are peeled and are about 3 inches long. They look so amazing in this dish.

Per serving: Calories: 83; Fat: 3g; Carbohydrates: 15g; Fiber: 3g; Protein: 1g; Sodium: 85mg; Vitamin B12: 0%; Iron: 2%

Molasses Cookies

Makes 2 dozen cookies

Prep time: 20 minutes / Cook time: 10 minutes

These gingery, cinnamony cookies are the perfect ending to any meal, not only because molasses has lower sugar content than most processed sugars. It also has the added bonus of being a source of calcium, iron, and magnesium.

¼ cup sugar

12 tablespoons (1½ sticks) butter or margarine

1 cup brown sugar

¼ cup molasses

1 large egg

2 cups all-purpose flour

2 teaspoons baking soda

1 teaspoon ground cinnamon

½ teaspoon ground ginger

Pinch ground cloves

Pinch salt

1. Preheat the oven to 375°F. Line a baking sheet with parchment paper. Put the sugar in a small bowl and set aside.
2. In a stand mixer fitted with the paddle attachment, beat the butter and brown sugar on medium speed until light and fluffy.
3. Add the molasses and egg and beat until well combined. With the mixer on low, add the flour, baking soda, cinnamon, ginger, cloves, and salt and mix until well combined.
4. Take about 2 tablespoons of dough and roll it into a 1-inch ball. Roll the ball in the sugar, and place it on the prepared baking sheet. Repeat with the rest of the dough, spacing the balls 2 inches apart. The cookies will spread while baking.
5. Bake for 8 to 10 minutes. Let cool on a wire rack.
6. The cookies can be stored in an airtight container at room temperature for up to 5 days or frozen for up to 3 months.

Per serving (1 cookie): Calories: 128; Fat: 6g; Carbohydrates: 20g; Fiber: <1g; Protein: 1g; Sodium: 156mg; Vitamin B12: 1%; Iron: 4%

Mini Cheesecakes

Makes 12 cheesecakes

Prep time: 15 minutes / Cook time: 25 minutes

You can't beat an indulgent dessert that's rich enough to make you forget you're on a special diet. The cream cheese at the center of this dessert is a low-residue staple, and the cook time is low thanks to the muffin tin the cakes are baked in. Bring these itty-bitty cheesecakes to a dinner party—everyone loves cheesecake!

1 cup graham cracker crumbs or Oreo cookie crumbs

3 tablespoons butter or margarine, at room temperature

2 (8-ounce) packages cream cheese, at room temperature

½ cup sugar

1 teaspoon vanilla extract

½ teaspoon lemon juice

2 large eggs

1. Preheat the oven to 350°F. Place muffin liners in a 12-cup muffin tin.
2. In a medium bowl, mix together the graham cracker crumbs and butter. Press the mixture equally into the lined muffin cups.
3. Bake for 5 minutes. Let cool on a wire rack.
4. Using a hand mixer, stand mixer, or whisk, mix together the cream cheese, sugar, vanilla, lemon juice, and eggs until smooth. Divide the mixture equally among the 12 muffin cups.
5. Bake for 18 to 20 minutes, or until the cheesecakes are set.
6. Let cool on a wire rack. Peel off the muffin liners before serving.
7. Store these cheesecakes in an airtight container in the refrigerator for up to 5 days or freeze them for up to 3 months.

Per serving (1 cheesecake): Calories: 229; Fat: 17g; Carbohydrates: 15g; Fiber: <1g; Protein: 4g; Sodium: 220mg; Vitamin B12: 4%; Iron: 5%

Mini Pineapple Upside-Down Cakes

Makes 12 cakes

Prep time: 15 minutes / Cook time: 30 minutes

These mini pineapple upside-down cakes are moist and not overly sweet but still so satisfying. The butter, sugar, and pineapple on top of the cakes give them a beautiful caramelized flavor and color.

12 tablespoons (1½ sticks) butter, at room temperature, divided

2 tablespoons sugar, plus ½ cup

12 pineapple rings, fresh or canned

1½ cups all-purpose flour

1 teaspoon baking powder

Pinch salt

1 large egg

¼ cup milk of choice

¼ cup sour cream or plain Greek yogurt

1 teaspoon vanilla extract

1. Preheat the oven to 350°F. Spray a 12-cup muffin tin with cooking spray.
2. Place 1 teaspoon of butter in each muffin cup. Sprinkle ½ teaspoon of sugar into each muffin cup.
3. Trim the pineapple rings to fit the bottom of the muffin cups and place in the bottom of each one, reserving the trimmed pieces.
4. In a large bowl, mix together the flour, baking powder, and salt and set aside.
5. In a stand mixer with the paddle attachment, beat the remaining 8 tablespoons of butter and the remaining ½ cup of sugar until light and creamy. Add the egg, milk, sour cream, and vanilla and beat until smooth.
6. Add the flour mixture, ¼ cup at a time, and beat until smooth.
7. Chop the remaining pineapple into small pieces and gently fold them into the batter.

continued ▸

Mini Pineapple Upside-Down Cakes continued

8. Spoon the batter equally into the 12 muffin cups.
9. Bake for 25 to 30 minutes, or until a toothpick inserted into one of the cakes comes out clean. Let the cakes cool in the pan for 5 minutes.
10. Place a large cutting board over the muffin tin and carefully flip them both over to release the cakes from the pan. Let cool and serve.

Per serving (1 cake): Calories: 241; Fat: 13g; Carbohydrates: 29g; Fiber: 2g; Protein: 3g; Sodium: 140mg; Vitamin B12: 2%; Iron: 5%

Dark Chocolate Mug Cake

Serves 1

Prep time: 5 minutes / Cook time: 2 minutes

Do you ever crave chocolate cake but fear you might end up eating too much (and inadvertently intensifying some of your symptoms)? This mug cake is the perfect compromise. It makes 1 delicious serving of decadent chocolate cake that is ready in less than 10 minutes. Just enough to curb your craving.

¼ cup dark chocolate chips
1 teaspoon canola or vegetable oil
1 large egg
½ cup milk of choice
4 tablespoons all-purpose flour
3 tablespoons brown sugar
2 tablespoons unsweetened dark cocoa powder
¼ teaspoon vanilla extract

1. In a large mug, mix together the dark chocolate chips and oil. Heat in the microwave in 20-second intervals until the chocolate melts. Let cool.
2. Add the egg, milk, flour, brown sugar, cocoa powder, and vanilla and stir until well combined.
3. Heat in the microwave oven for 1 to 1½ minutes, or until the top is cooked but the middle is still gooey.

low-residue

Per serving: Calories: 668; Fat: 30g; Carbohydrates: 107g; Fiber: 9g; Protein: 15g; Sodium: 286mg; Vitamin B12: 17%; Iron: 33%

Black Bean Burgers . page 120

6.

High-Fiber Recipes

Breakfast

Entrées

continued ▸

High-Fiber Recipes

continued

Sides

Desserts

Chocolate–Peanut Butter Smoothie Bowls

Serves 4

Prep time: 10 minutes

Three tablespoons of unsweetened dark cocoa powder has 5 grams of fiber and 15 percent of your daily recommended iron intake. Not bad for something that makes food taste so good. This smoothie bowl can be a quick, 5-minute breakfast or an opportunity to flex your creativity when you're not in a hurry. Delicious, beautiful, and packed with healthy fats, fiber, and iron. What's not to love?

3 frozen bananas

½ cup diced avocado

2 cups plain Greek yogurt

1½ cups milk of choice

3 tablespoons peanut butter

3 tablespoons unsweetened dark cocoa powder

1 tablespoon chia seeds

1 tablespoon ground flaxseed

1 teaspoon vanilla extract

OPTIONAL TOPPINGS

Fresh fruit

Chia seeds

Hemp seeds

Shredded coconut flakes

Granola

Nuts of choice

1. Place the bananas, avocado, yogurt, milk, peanut butter, cocoa powder, chia, flaxseed, and vanilla into a blender and puree until smooth.
2. Pour into bowls and garnish with the optional toppings.

Per serving: Calories: 366; Fat: 17g; Carbohydrates: 38g; Fiber: 7g; Protein: 20g; Sodium: 188mg; Vitamin B12: 7%; Iron: 12%

Strawberry-Banana Breakfast Parfait

Serves 4

Prep time: 15 minutes

This parfait uses Greek yogurt, which has more protein than regular yogurt. Thanks to the strawberries and bananas, this parfait is sweet without being high in sugar.

2 cups plain Greek yogurt

2 tablespoons honey or maple syrup

½ teaspoon ground cinnamon

½ teaspoon vanilla extract

2 cups no-added-sugar muesli or uncooked oats (see Helpful Hints)

1 tablespoon chia seeds

1 tablespoon pumpkin seeds

2 cups sliced strawberries

1 banana, sliced

1. In a small bowl, mix together the yogurt, honey, cinnamon, and vanilla.
2. Spoon ¼ cup of the yogurt mixture into the bottom of a drinking glass. Top with ¼ cup of the muesli and a thin layer of chia and pumpkin seeds, and sprinkle with strawberry and banana slices. Repeat the layers until the glass is full. Repeat with the rest of the ingredients. Serve immediately.

Helpful Hints: If using uncooked oats, refrigerate the parfaits overnight to give the oats time to soften. Otherwise, they'll be tough and chewy.

Try these alternate flavor combinations instead of the strawberries and banana:
Berry: 1 cup sliced strawberries, ½ cup raspberries, and ½ cup blueberries
Piña colada: 1 cup diced pineapple and 2 tablespoons coconut flakes
Cherry cheesecake: 1 cup cherries and 2 tablespoons cream cheese

---

Per serving: Calories: 384; Fat: 11g; Carbohydrates: 60g; Fiber: 8g; Protein: 17g; Sodium: 145mg; Vitamin B12: 0%; Iron: 12%

Breakfast Ice Cream

Serves 4

Prep time: 10 minutes

With this recipe, you can indulge your craving for ice cream and embrace your inner child at breakfast without sacrificing your nutrition. Not only is it packed with fiber, vitamins, and minerals, if you pair it with a source of protein, such as eggs or Greek yogurt (and I recommend that you do), it will help keep you full. Try using a tropical blend of pineapples and mangos for a change of pace.

2 cups frozen raspberries or blackberries

4 frozen bananas

½ avocado

¼ cup unsweetened applesauce

1 tablespoon chia seeds

1 tablespoon honey or maple syrup, plus more as needed

Combine the berries, bananas, avocado, applesauce, chia seeds, and honey in a food processor or blender and process until smooth. (It should be the consistency of soft-serve ice cream.) Taste and add more honey if needed. Serve immediately.

Helpful Hint: It's probably not a surprise that this ice cream freezes well. Make it ahead of time so you'll have a quick breakfast in the morning or if you prefer your ice cream on the firmer side.

Per serving: Calories: 214; Fat: 5g; Carbohydrates: 45g; Fiber: 11g; Protein: 4g; Sodium: 4mg; Vitamin B12: 0%; Iron: 5%

Apple-Cinnamon Baked Oatmeal Squares

Makes 9 squares

Prep time: 10 minutes / Cook time: 35 minutes

The perfect make-ahead breakfast, these oatmeal squares are packed with fiber to help keep you full throughout the morning—and symptoms at bay. They taste like apple crumble, and they smell like it, too—the aromas will fill the house. Make these in preparation for travel, camping, or just running errands.

1½ cups milk
2 large eggs
½ cup brown sugar
½ cup unsweetened applesauce
4 tablespoons (½ stick) butter, melted
2 teaspoons ground cinnamon
1½ teaspoons baking powder
1 teaspoon vanilla extract
Pinch salt
3 cups rolled oats
2 apples, Honey Crisp, Fuji, Granny Smith, or Gala, peeled and finely diced
1 tablespoon chia seeds
2¼ cups plain or vanilla Greek yogurt

1. Preheat the oven to 350°F.
2. In a large mixing bowl, whisk together the milk, eggs, brown sugar, applesauce, butter, cinnamon, baking powder, vanilla, and salt until well combined.
3. Add the oats, apples, and chia seeds and mix to incorporate.
4. Pour the oatmeal mixture into an 8-by-8-inch baking dish and spread out evenly. Bake for 30 to 35 minutes, or until the oatmeal is set. Let cool on a wire rack for 5 minutes.
5. Cut into 9 squares and serve with ¼ cup of Greek yogurt each for a complete meal.

Per serving (1 square): Calories: 293; Fat: 12g; Carbohydrates: 40g; Fiber: 4g; Protein: 12g; Sodium: 183mg; Vitamin B12: 5%; Iron: 11%

Overnight Steel-Cut Oats

Serves 4

Prep time: 5 minutes, plus 4 hours chilling time

Overnight oats are the pinnacle of stress-free meals—they let the refrigerator do all the work. These oats are easily customizable, so play with the different flavor options.

FOR THE OATS

- 1 cup steel-cut oats
- ⅔ cup milk or nondairy milk of choice
- 1 tablespoon chia seeds
- 1 tablespoon hemp seeds
- 1 teaspoon ground cinnamon

FLAVOR OPTIONS

BERRY

- 1 cup frozen berries of choice

PUMPKIN SPICE

- 1 tablespoon canned pumpkin puree
- 1 teaspoon ground cinnamon
- Pinch nutmeg

TROPICAL

- 1 tablespoon shredded coconut
- 1 cup pineapple, diced
- 1 cup mango, diced

PEACH COBBLER

- 1 cup canned peaches packed in water
- Pinch ground cinnamon

PEANUT BUTTER-BANANA

- 1 banana, chopped
- 2 tablespoons peanut butter

APPLE PIE

- 2 apples, Honey Crisp, Fuji, Granny Smith, or Gala, chopped, or 4 tablespoons unsweetened applesauce
- ½ teaspoon ground cinnamon
- Handful pecans

1. In a medium airtight container, mix together the oats, milk, chia, hemp, and cinnamon. Gently stir in the toppings of your choice, cover, and refrigerate for at least 4 hours or overnight.
2. Serve cold, but if you prefer your oats hot, place them in a microwave-safe bowl and heat them in the microwave for 2 to 3 minutes, or place them in a small saucepan over low heat until warmed through.

Helpful Hints: Store oats and hemp seeds in a cool, dry place or in the freezer to extend their shelf life.

Per serving for the oats: Calories: 188; Fat: 5g; Carbohydrates: 31g; Fiber: 6g; Protein: 9g; Sodium: 18mg; Vitamin B12: 3%; Iron: 15%

High-Fiber Bran Muffins

Makes 12 muffins

Prep time: 10 minutes / Cook time: 18 minutes

At less than 30 minutes from start to finish, this recipe is great for busy weekdays. I always have a dozen muffins stored in the freezer to pull out for a quick, nutritious morning bite.

1 cup wheat bran

1 cup whole-wheat flour

¾ cup sugar

2 teaspoons baking powder

1 teaspoon baking soda

1 teaspoon ground cinnamon

½ teaspoon salt

1 large egg

1 cup plain Greek yogurt

½ cup canola oil

1 tablespoon chia seeds

½ cup berries of choice

1. Preheat the oven to 375°F. Place muffin liners in a 12-cup muffin tin.
2. In a large bowl, mix together the wheat bran, flour, sugar, baking powder, baking soda, cinnamon, and salt. Set aside.
3. In a small bowl, whisk together the egg, yogurt, canola oil, and chia seeds.
4. Form a well in the center of the dry ingredients. Pour the yogurt mixture into it and mix just until incorporated. Be careful not to overmix, or the muffins will be tough.
5. Fold in the berries. Divide the batter evenly among the muffin cups.
6. Bake for 15 to 18 minutes, or until a toothpick inserted into the center of a muffin comes out clean.
7. The muffins can be stored in an airtight container at room temperature for up to 5 days or frozen for up to 3 months.

Helpful Hint: Instead of berries, add 1 cup grated carrot and ¼ cup raisins, or for that chocolate lover in the house, ½ cup dark chocolate chips.

Per serving: Calories: 206; Fat: 11g; Carbohydrates: 24g; Fiber: 4g; Protein: 5g; Sodium: 296mg; Vitamin B12: 1%; Iron: 7%

Almond-Orange Cranberry Loaf

Makes 1 loaf (12 servings)
Prep time: 10 minutes / Cook time: 55 minutes

Packed with vitamin C and fiber, cranberries are powerful little berries—a great choice for managing your symptoms.

2 cups whole-wheat flour
1 teaspoon ground cinnamon
1 teaspoon baking powder
½ teaspoon baking soda
⅓ cup sugar
4 tablespoons (½ stick) butter or margarine, at room temperature
2 large eggs
1 cup freshly squeezed orange juice
1 cup dried unsweetened cranberries
¾ cup sliced almonds
2 tablespoons chia seeds
1 teaspoon orange zest

1. Preheat the oven to 350°F. Grease a 5-by-9-inch loaf pan and set aside.
2. In a large bowl, combine the flour, cinnamon, baking powder, and baking soda. Set aside.
3. In a separate bowl, whisk together the sugar and butter until light and fluffy. Add the eggs one at a time, whisking well to incorporate. Add the orange juice and whisk until well mixed.
4. Form a well in the center of the dry ingredients. Add the sugar mixture and fold in using a rubber spatula. Add the cranberries, almonds, chia, and orange zest and fold into the batter. Be careful not to overmix, or the loaf will be tough.
5. Pour the batter into the prepared loaf pan and spread out evenly. Bake for 50 to 55 minutes, or until a toothpick inserted into the center comes out clean.
6. Let cool in the pan on a wire rack for 10 minutes. Remove the loaf from the pan and cool completely before serving.

Per serving: Calories: 187; Fat: 6g; Carbohydrates: 29g; Fiber: 3g; Protein: 4g; Sodium: 229mg; Vitamin B12: 2%; Iron: 8%

Gingerbread Pancakes

Serves 4

Prep time: 15 minutes / Cook time: 25 minutes

These pancakes are a spiced twist on the classic breakfast staple, but I've snuck in lentils for a healthy dose of protein and fiber. (Don't worry—you'll never know they are there.)

- **½ cup whole-wheat flour**
- **¼ cup sugar**
- **1½ teaspoons baking powder**
- **½ teaspoon baking soda**
- **½ teaspoon salt**
- **1 cup canned lentils, rinsed**
- **2 large eggs**
- **¼ cup molasses**
- **¼ cup milk of choice**
- **3 tablespoons canola oil**
- **1 teaspoon ground ginger**
- **1 teaspoon ground cinnamon**
- **½ teaspoon ground cloves**
- **1 teaspoon vegetable oil or cooking spray**

1. In a medium bowl, sift together the flour, sugar, baking powder, baking soda, and salt. Set aside.
2. Place the lentils in a blender or food processor and puree until completely smooth. Add water 1 tablespoon at a time to thin enough to puree.
3. In a separate large bowl, whisk together the eggs, molasses, milk, canola oil, ginger, cinnamon, and cloves.
4. Mix the flour mixture into the lentil mixture and stir until smooth.
5. Set a large sauté pan or skillet over medium heat. Lightly grease with the vegetable oil. Spoon ¼ cup of batter into the skillet and cook until bubbles start to form around the edges, 2 to 3 minutes. Flip and cook until golden brown, another 2 to 3 minutes. Serve with desired toppings.
6. Store leftovers in the refrigerator for up to 5 days or in the freezer for up to 4 months. To reheat, heat in the microwave until hot.

Per serving: Calories: 365; Fat: 15g; Carbohydrates: 49g; Fiber: 6g; Protein: 10g; Sodium: 683mg; Vitamin B12: 5%; Iron: 23%

Quinoa and Avocado Scramble

Serves 4

Prep time: 10 minutes / Cook time: 20 minutes

Start your day off right with this protein-packed breakfast. Quinoa is the only grain that is a complete protein, with 14.1 grams of protein per cup, and it's high in fiber to boot. Be sure to rinse the quinoa before cooking it, as the seed's natural coating can have a bitter or soapy flavor, though some brands come pre-rinsed.

⅓ cup quinoa, rinsed
⅔ cup water
1 teaspoon vegetable oil
2 green onions, chopped
1 red bell pepper, diced
Salt
Freshly ground black pepper
4 large eggs, beaten
½ cup shredded Cheddar cheese
¼ cup chunky salsa
1 ripe avocado, peeled, pitted, and cut into slices
2 tablespoons fresh lime juice

1. In a medium saucepan over high heat, mix together the quinoa and water and bring to a boil. Lower the heat to medium, cover, and continue to cook until the water is absorbed, about 15 minutes. Set aside.
2. In a large saucepan over medium heat, warm the oil until it just begins to shimmer. Add the green onions and peppers and cook until the vegetables begin to brown, 1 to 2 minutes. Lightly season with salt and pepper.
3. Add the eggs and cook, stirring often, until cooked through, 1 to 2 minutes. Remove from the heat.
4. Divide the quinoa equally among four bowls. Top with equal amounts of the egg mixture, shredded cheese, salsa, avocado slices, and a drizzle of lime juice. Serve hot.

Per serving: Calories: 283; Fat: 18g; Carbohydrates: 18g; Fiber: 5g; Protein: 12g; Sodium: 291mg; Vitamin B12: 8%; Iron: 11%

Vegetarian Breakfast Burritos

Serves 6

Prep time: 10 minutes / Cook time: 10 minutes

Breakfast burritos are one of my favorite recipes, mostly because they're so easy to make ahead and freeze for later. Here I've packed them with delicious veggies and black beans, but if you prefer even more flavor, add some chopped fresh cilantro or a dash of hot sauce. Whole-grain tortillas have more fiber than whole-wheat or regular flour tortillas, so look for them at your grocery store.

1 tablespoon canola oil
3 cups canned black beans, drained and rinsed
2 tomatoes, diced
2 bell peppers, diced
1 cup chopped fresh spinach
1 bunch green onions, chopped
6 large eggs, beaten
Salt
Freshly ground black pepper
6 whole-grain tortillas
1 cup shredded Cheddar cheese
1 avocado, diced
6 tablespoons salsa, for serving
6 tablespoons plain Greek yogurt, for serving

1. In a large pan over medium heat, warm the oil until it just begins to shimmer.
2. Add the beans, tomatoes, bell peppers, spinach, and green onions and cook until the vegetables begin to brown and become fragrant, about 2 minutes.
3. Add the eggs and cook, stirring, until the eggs are cooked and are no longer runny, 1 to 2 minutes. Season with salt and pepper to taste.
4. Divide the egg mixture equally among the tortillas, keeping the filling in a line near the middle of the tortilla. Sprinkle with the shredded cheese and diced avocado.
5. To wrap the burritos, take the left and right sides of the tortilla and fold them inward. Take the bottom side and fold it up and over the filling, rolling to wrap it up completely. Repeat with the remaining burritos.

6. Serve warm with 1 tablespoon each of salsa and Greek yogurt per burrito.

7. Store the burritos, wrapped in plastic wrap, in the refrigerator for up to 5 days or in the freezer for up to 3 months. To reheat, defrost frozen burritos in the refrigerator overnight and heat in the microwave or in a 350°F oven until hot, if you like a crispier burrito.

Helpful Hint: Try a salt-free seasoning like Mrs. Dash to add a pop of flavor.

Per serving (1 burrito): Calories: 497; Fat: 22g; Carbohydrates: 53g; Fiber: 12g; Protein: 24g; Sodium: 557mg; Vitamin B12: 8%; Iron: 16%

Minestrone Soup

Serves 4

Prep time: 15 minutes / Cook time: 35 minutes

Minestrone is a thick Italian soup that is packed with fiber and is usually made with whatever vegetables are on hand.

- 1 cup high-fiber small pasta shells
- 1 teaspoon canola or vegetable oil
- ½ white or Spanish onion, diced
- 2 celery stalks, diced
- 1 garlic clove, minced
- 1 tablespoon Italian seasoning
- 6 cups vegetable stock
- 1 (28-ounce) can diced tomatoes
- 1 tablespoon tomato paste
- 1 (15-ounce) can kidney beans, drained and rinsed
- 1 cup frozen mixed carrots and green beans
- Salt
- Freshly ground black pepper
- Freshly grated Parmesan cheese (optional)

1. Bring a large saucepan of water to a boil over high heat and cook the pasta according to the package instructions until al dente, about 8 minutes. Drain, transfer to a bowl, and set aside.
2. In a large stockpot over medium heat, warm the oil. Add the onion, celery, garlic, and Italian seasoning and cook until the onions are translucent, about 4 minutes. Raise the heat to medium-high. Add the vegetable stock, diced tomatoes, and tomato paste and bring to a boil. Lower the heat to medium-low, cover, and simmer, stirring occasionally, for 15 to 20 minutes.
3. Add the kidney beans, frozen mixed carrots and green beans, and cooked pasta, and continue to simmer until heated through, about 5 minutes. Season with salt and pepper as desired. Spoon into bowls, garnish with grated Parmesan (if using), and serve.
4. Store leftover soup in an airtight container in the refrigerator for up to 5 days or in the freezer for up to 3 months.

Per serving: Calories: 320; Fat: 2g; Carbohydrates: 63g; Fiber: 14g; Protein: 13g; Sodium: 1,067mg; Vitamin B12: 0%; Iron: 18%

Creamy Potato Soup

Serves 4

Prep time: 15 minutes / Cook time: 35 minutes

Potato may be the star of this dish, but it's the white beans that offer the benefits of increased fiber and protein that help keep you full. The beans are also packed with thiamin, folate, iron, magnesium, phosphorus, potassium, copper, and manganese, making this soup healthy for just about anyone. It's a great choice for feeding a crowd or your very hungry family.

3 cups chicken stock

4 russet potatoes, scrubbed and cut into small dice (with skin on)

2 teaspoons onion powder

1 teaspoon garlic powder

1 (15½-ounce) can white kidney beans, drained and rinsed

1 bunch green onions, chopped, divided

1½ cups shredded Cheddar cheese, divided

½ cup milk of choice

Salt

Freshly ground black pepper

1. In a large stockpot over medium-high heat, mix together the stock, potatoes, onion powder, and garlic powder and bring to a boil. Lower the heat to medium-low and simmer until the potatoes are cooked through, 15 to 20 minutes.
2. In a blender or food processor, puree the beans until smooth. If the mixture is too thick to blend, add water, 1 tablespoon at a time. Set aside.
3. Using an immersion blender, blend the potatoes until your desired consistency. I like mine to have a bit of texture, so I blend only half of the potatoes. Other family members like theirs silky smooth, and they blend smooth.
4. Stir the white bean puree into the potatoes and cook over low heat until heated through, about 15 minutes.

continued ▸

Creamy Potato Soup *continued*

5. Reserve 1 tablespoon of the chopped green onions and 2 tablespoons of the shredded cheese and set aside. Add the remaining green onions, the milk, and the remaining cheese to the soup and stir to combine.
6. Spoon into bowls and serve hot with the reserved green onions and cheese sprinkled over the top for garnish.
7. Leftover soup can be stored in an airtight container in the refrigerator for up to 5 days.

Helpful Hint: If you would like to freeze the soup, make the recipe as instructed, but leave out the milk. Freeze in airtight containers for up to 3 months. To reheat, let it thaw overnight in the refrigerator before placing it in a large saucepan over medium heat. Add the milk and cook, stirring occasionally, until heated through.

Per serving: Calories: 398; Fat: 14g; Carbohydrates: 50g; Fiber: 10g; Protein: 21g; Sodium: 728mg; Vitamin B12: 2%; Iron: 17%

Turkey Chili

Serves 4

Prep time: 15 minutes / Cook time: 35 minutes

Store-bought chili is packed with salt and saturated fats and tends to be low in vegetables. This homemade chili is made leaner by using ground turkey and lots of high-fiber beans and vegetables.

1 pound lean ground turkey, formed into a large patty

1 white or Spanish onion, diced

1 cup diced celery

2 garlic cloves, minced

2 tablespoons chili powder

1 tablespoon ground cumin

Pinch crushed red chili flakes

1 red or orange bell pepper, seeded and diced

1 cup sliced button mushrooms

1 (15-ounce) can baked beans in molasses

1 (15-ounce) can no-salt-added kidney beans, drained and rinsed

1 (15-ounce) can no-salt-added diced tomatoes

1 (6-ounce) can tomato paste

Salt

Freshly ground black pepper

1. In a large saucepan over medium heat, place the turkey patty. Cook until the meat browns, about 4 minutes. Flip the turkey and cook until browned, another 4 minutes. Using a spatula, break up the meat into small pieces.
2. Add the onion, celery, garlic, chili powder, cumin, and chili flakes and cook for 2 to 3 minutes.
3. Raise the heat to medium-high, add the bell pepper, mushrooms, baked beans, kidney beans, tomatoes, and tomato paste, and bring to a boil. Lower the heat to medium-low and simmer, stirring frequently to prevent burning, for 15 to 20 minutes. Taste and season with salt and pepper. Serve warm.
4. Store leftovers in an airtight container in the refrigerator for up to 5 days or in the freezer for up to 4 months.

Per serving: Calories: 499; Fat: 10g; Carbohydrates: 67g; Fiber: 21g; Protein: 40g; Sodium: 869mg; Vitamin B12: <1%; Iron: 54%

Jambalaya

Serves 6

Prep time: 10 minutes / Cook time: 40 minutes

Jambalaya originated in Louisiana, a state with Spanish, French, and West African influences. Most jambalayas start with the "holy trinity"—a mixture of onion, celery, and green bell pepper that is the foundation of Creole and Cajun cooking. Although most jambalayas use sausage, pork, chicken, and shrimp, this recipe includes just shrimp and chicken because diverticulitis sufferers should eat red meat sparingly.

3 teaspoons vegetable oil, divided

½ pound large shrimp, peeled and deveined

1 boneless, skinless chicken breast, cut into small pieces

5 celery stalks, chopped

3 green bell peppers, diced

½ white or Spanish onion, diced

1 garlic clove, minced

2 tablespoons Cajun seasoning

1½ cups Homemade Chicken Stock (page 61) or store-bought

1 cup brown basmati rice, rinsed

1 cup canned crushed tomatoes

Salt

Freshly ground black pepper

1. In a large saucepan over medium heat, warm 2 teaspoons of oil. Add the shrimp and cook until pink and golden, 1 to 2 minutes per side. Transfer the shrimp to a plate and set aside.
2. Add the chicken and cook until golden, cooked through, and no longer pink, about 5 minutes. Transfer the chicken to a plate and set aside.
3. Add the remaining 1 teaspoon of oil to the saucepan and warm until just shimmering. Add the celery, bell pepper, onion, garlic, and Cajun seasoning and cook until the onions are translucent, about 3 minutes.

4. Raise the heat to medium-high, add the chicken stock, rice, and crushed tomatoes, and bring to a boil. Lower the heat to medium-low and simmer for 20 to 25 minutes, or until the rice is cooked.
5. Stir in the chicken and shrimp. Taste and season with salt and pepper.
6. Store the jambalaya in an airtight container in the refrigerator for up to 5 days.

Helpful Hint: This dish actually tastes even better the next day as the flavors start to grow.

Per serving: Calories: 226; Fat: 5g; Carbohydrates: 32g; Fiber: 4g; Protein: 17g; Sodium: 1,418mg; Vitamin B12: 7%; Iron: 12%

Taco Salad

Serves 4

Prep time: 15 minutes / Cook time: 15 minutes

This entrée salad is totally customizable to your veggie preferences. Making it with ground turkey or chicken instead of beef decreases your chances of a flare-up.

1 teaspoon vegetable oil

½ pound lean ground turkey or ground chicken, formed into a large patty

2 tablespoons taco seasoning (see Helpful Hint)

Salt

Freshly ground black pepper

6 cups chopped romaine lettuce

Toppings

2 red or orange bell peppers, diced

3 Roma tomatoes, diced

½ English cucumber, diced

¾ cup green onions, thinly sliced

1 (15½-ounce) can black beans, rinsed and drained

Salsa

Sour cream or plain Greek yogurt

1. In a large sauté pan or skillet over medium heat, warm the oil. Add the turkey patty and cook until browned, about 4 minutes. Flip the turkey and cook until browned, another 4 minutes. Use a spatula to break up the turkey into small pieces. Add the taco seasoning, stir to combine, and cook until completely cooked through, another 5 minutes. Taste, and season with salt and pepper.
2. Place the romaine lettuce in individual bowls. Spoon the taco meat over the lettuce.
3. Place the toppings in individual bowls and set out at the table. Diners can choose whichever toppings they like.

Helpful Hint: If you don't have taco seasoning, use a mixture of 1 tablespoon chili powder, 1 teaspoon ground cumin, 1 teaspoon garlic powder, 1 teaspoon onion powder, and a pinch crushed red chili flakes.

Per serving: Calories: 265; Fat: 7g; Carbohydrates: 33g; Fiber: 10g; Protein: 21g; Sodium: 273mg; Vitamin B12: 0%; Iron: 25%

Santa Fe Cobb Salad

Serves 4

Prep time: 25 minutes / Cook time: 7 minutes

For a hearty salad you can eat as a meal on its own, you've come to the right place. Corn was once thought to aggravate the symptoms of diverticulitis, but newer research has found that eating modest amounts of corn will not make your condition worse (but moderation is the key!).

4 slices bacon

6 cups chopped romaine lettuce

4 hard-boiled eggs, sliced

2 avocados, sliced

1½ cups cherry tomatoes, halved

1 cup canned or frozen roasted corn

1 cup shelled edamame or canned black beans, rinsed and drained

½ cup diced red onion

4 ounces crumbled goat cheese

Ranch, blue cheese, or chipotle ranch dressing

Hot sauce

1. Line a plate with paper towels. In a large sauté pan or skillet over medium heat, cook the bacon until crisp, 5 to 7 minutes. Transfer the bacon to the lined plate. When cool, crumble the bacon into bits and set aside.
2. Divide the romaine between four bowls.
3. Arrange the eggs, avocados, tomatoes, corn, edamame, onion, goat cheese, and bacon bits in neat lines over the lettuce.
4. Lightly drizzle with the desired dressing and a splash of hot sauce.

Helpful Hint: The salads can be made ahead of time and kept in airtight containers so you'll have quick lunches or dinners to accommodate a busy work week. Be sure to use a plastic or nylon knife to cut the lettuce or tear the leaves with your hands to keep them from browning. I like to put the dressing in a small container on the side to keep the salad from getting soggy.

Per serving: Calories: 463; Fat: 30g; Carbohydrates: 29g; Fiber: 10g; Protein: 25g; Sodium: 385mg; Vitamin B12: 12%; Iron: 22%

Stuffed Sweet Potatoes

Serves 4

Prep time: 10 minutes / Cook time: 1 hour

What's better than a stuffed potato? A stuffed sweet potato! When baked, sweet potatoes have twice the amount of fiber as white potatoes, making this recipe a good alternative to traditional baked potatoes when you are trying to avoid flare-ups. This is also gluten-free, which is a nice option for people with allergies.

2 cups quinoa, rinsed
1⅓ cups water
4 medium sweet potatoes, scrubbed
1 tablespoon vegetable oil
½ red onion, diced
4 cups fresh spinach
1 red bell pepper, diced
1 cup diced zucchini
1 garlic clove, minced
1 (15½-ounce) can chickpeas, drained and rinsed
Salt
Freshly ground black pepper
2 tablespoons tahini
1 tablespoon lemon juice
Pinch ground cumin
4 Roma tomatoes, diced
1 cup crumbled feta cheese

1. In a medium saucepan over high heat, mix together the quinoa and water and bring to a boil. Lower the heat to medium, cover, and continue to cook until the water is absorbed, about 15 minutes. Set aside.
2. Preheat the oven to 400°F. Line a baking sheet with parchment paper.
3. Pierce the sweet potatoes with a fork several times and place them on the prepared baking sheet. Bake for 35 to 45 minutes, or until a knife inserted into a sweet potato meets no resistance.
4. In a large sauté pan or skillet over medium heat, warm the oil. Add the red onion and cook until translucent, about 3 minutes. Add the spinach, red bell pepper, zucchini, and garlic and cook for 5 minutes.
5. Add the quinoa and chickpeas and stir to combine. Taste and season with salt and pepper. Set aside and keep warm.

6. In a small bowl, mix together the tahini, lemon juice, and cumin to make the dressing. If it is too thick to drizzle, thin it out with more lemon juice or water.

7. Cut the potatoes in half, about ¾ of the way through. Squeeze the ends to open them up a bit. Stuff the potatoes with the vegetable and quinoa mixture. Top with the feta cheese and diced tomatoes, and drizzle with the tahini dressing. Serve warm.

8. To store, wrap each stuffed potato individually in plastic wrap and refrigerate for up to 5 days.

Per serving: Calories: 811; Fat: 24g; Carbohydrates: 125g; Fiber: 17g; Protein: 28g; Sodium: 482mg; Vitamin B12: 11%; Iron: 55%

Vegetable Stir-Fry

Serves 6

Prep time: 15 minutes / Cook time: 25 minutes

Taste the rainbow in this super colorful stir-fry. Throw in any leftover veggies you have in your refrigerator, or add chicken or salmon.

¼ cup soy sauce
2 tablespoons sesame oil
1 tablespoon pineapple or orange juice
1 tablespoon cornstarch
1 cup brown rice
1¾ cups water
2 carrots, chopped
1 cup broccoli florets
1 cup cauliflower florets
2 teaspoons vegetable oil
1 small white or Spanish onion, thinly sliced
2 garlic cloves, minced
2 cups shelled edamame
1 cup quartered button mushrooms
1 cup sugar snap peas
1 bell pepper, diced

1. In a small bowl, mix together the soy sauce, sesame oil, pineapple juice, and cornstarch until smooth.
2. In a medium saucepan over high heat, mix the rice with the water and bring to a boil. Lower the heat to medium-low, cover, and cook for 10 minutes. Remove from the heat and let sit, covered, for an additional 10 minutes. Set aside.
3. Bring a medium saucepan of water to a boil over medium-high heat. Add the carrots, broccoli, and cauliflower and cook until tender-crisp, about 3 minutes. Drain and set aside.
4. In a large sauté pan or skillet over medium heat, warm the vegetable oil. Add the onion and cook for 3 minutes. Add the garlic, edamame, mushrooms, snap peas, bell pepper, carrots, broccoli, and cauliflower and cook until the vegetables are tender, about 5 minutes.
5. Pour the sauce over vegetables, stir, and cook for 5 more minutes.
6. Serve the stir-fry over the rice.

Per serving: Calories: 262; Fat: 8g; Carbohydrates: 39g; Fiber: 5g; Protein: 12g; Sodium: 672mg; Vitamin B12: <1%; Iron: 13%

Vegetarian Sushi Bowls

Serves 4

Prep time: 15 minutes / Cook time: 50 minutes

This bowl has all the flavors you love from your beloved Japanese restaurant—without the fish. If you are looking for a little crispy texture, add some roasted nori (seaweed) strips. Yum!

FOR THE RICE

1 cup brown rice

2½ cups water

2 tablespoons rice wine vinegar

2 tablespoons sugar

FOR THE TOPPINGS

1 English cucumber, thinly sliced

¼ cup thinly sliced radishes

1 avocado, sliced

1 cup shelled edamame

3 carrots, thinly sliced

2 green onions, finely chopped

2 teaspoons black sesame seeds, for garnish

1. Rinse the rice under warm water in a fine mesh sieve until the water runs clear. Place the rice in a medium saucepan over high heat, cover with the water, and bring to a boil. Lower the heat to medium-low, cover, and cook for 35 to 45 minutes, until all the water has been absorbed. Remove from the heat and let sit, covered, until ready to use.
2. In a small saucepan over medium-high heat, mix together the rice vinegar and sugar and cook until the sugar dissolves, about 5 minutes.
3. Pour the vinegar mixture over the rice and mix to combine.
4. Assemble the sushi bowls by spooning the rice into bowls and topping with the cucumber, radishes, avocado, edamame, carrots, and green onions. Sprinkle the black sesame seeds over the top and serve.
5. Store the assembled bowls covered with plastic wrap in the refrigerator for up to 5 days.

Per serving: Calories: 345; Fat: 10g; Carbohydrates: 57g; Fiber: 8g; Protein: 11g; Sodium: 74mg; Vitamin B12: 0%; Iron: 13%

High-Fiber Mac and Cheese

Serves 4 to 6

Prep time: 15 minutes / Cook time: 20 minutes

This healthier alternative to macaroni and cheese is loaded with fiber, protein, folate, iron, and calcium. It will surely keep you satisfied!

- **2½ cups whole-wheat or high-fiber elbow macaroni**
- **1 tablespoon olive oil**
- **1 cup canned brown or green lentils, rinsed, drained**
- **3 tablespoons butter or margarine**
- **3 tablespoons all-purpose flour**
- **1 teaspoon onion powder**
- **¼ teaspoon Dijon mustard**
- **Pinch ground nutmeg**
- **1¾ cups half-and-half or whipping cream**
- **1½ cups shredded sharp Cheddar cheese**
- **Salt**
- **Freshly ground black pepper**

1. Bring a large saucepan of water to a boil over high heat and cook the macaroni until al dente, according to the package instructions, about 8 minutes. Drain the pasta and toss with the olive oil to prevent the noodles from sticking.
2. Puree the lentils in a blender or food processor until smooth. If the mixture is too thick, add water 1 tablespoon at a time and continue to puree until smooth. Set aside.
3. In a large saucepan over medium heat, melt the butter. Add the flour, onion powder, Dijon mustard, and nutmeg, and cook, stirring constantly, for 1 minute. Slowly whisk in the half-and-half and bring to a boil. Lower the heat to medium-low and simmer, whisking constantly, for 2 minutes.
4. Remove from the heat, add the lentil puree and shredded cheese, and stir until the cheese is melted. Taste and season with salt and pepper. Add the macaroni to the sauce and stir until completely combined. Serve hot.

Per serving: Calories: 751; Fat: 40g; Carbohydrates: 72g; Fiber: 10g; Protein: 26g; Sodium: 383mg; Vitamin B12: 6%; Iron: 24%

Lentil Curry

Serves 4

Prep time: 10 minutes / Cook time: 1 hour 15 minutes

Curry is a seasoning made up of a variety of spices, typically including ginger, turmeric, cumin, coriander, and chili powder or cayenne. Curry powder ingredients will change from brand to brand, so each one will have a slightly different flavor. Garam masala is made with similar spices to curry powder, but it also has cinnamon, cardamom, nutmeg, cloves, bay leaves, peppercorn, fennel, mace, and chiles. I've included both curry and garam masala in this recipe, which will lend their intense flavors to the high-fiber lentils.

- 1½ cups brown basmati rice
- 2½ cups cold water
- 2 teaspoons vegetable oil
- 1 white or Spanish onion, diced small
- 1 garlic clove, minced
- 2 tablespoons curry powder
- 1 teaspoon garam masala
- 1 cup dried red lentils, rinsed
- 2½ cups vegetable or chicken stock
- 1 (6-ounce) can tomato paste
- 1 cup coconut milk
- 1 teaspoon soy sauce
- ½ teaspoon lime juice
- ½ teaspoon honey
- Salt
- Freshly ground black pepper
- ½ cup plain Greek yogurt

1. Rinse the rice in cold water until the water runs clear. Place the rice and water in a medium saucepan over high heat and bring to a boil. Lower the heat to medium-low, cover, and simmer for 50 minutes. Remove from the heat and let sit, covered, for 5 minutes. Fluff with a fork and set aside.
2. In a large sauté pan or skillet over medium heat, warm the oil. Add the onions, garlic, curry powder, and garam masala and cook until the onions are translucent, about 3 minutes. Add the lentils and cook for another 2 minutes. Raise the heat to medium-high, add the stock and tomato paste, and bring to a boil. Lower the heat to medium-low and simmer for 10 to 15 minutes.

continued ▸

Lentil Curry continued

3. Add the coconut milk, soy sauce, lime juice, and honey, stir to combine, and simmer for 5 minutes. Taste and season with salt and pepper. Garnish with a dollop of plain Greek yogurt.

4. Serve hot over the brown rice.

Helpful Hint: If you prefer a spicier curry, add cayenne pepper or hot sauce along with the coconut milk.

Per serving: Calories: 641; Fat: 18g; Carbohydrates: 100g; Fiber: 12g; Protein: 23g; Sodium: 786mg; Vitamin B12: 0%; Iron: 44%

Farro Risotto

Serves 4

Prep time: 10 minutes / Cook time: 20 minutes

Farro is an ancient grain with a nutty flavor and chewy texture that is commonly grown in the Tuscany region of Italy. This recipe is a modern, high-fiber spin on risotto, the classic Italian dish usually made with arborio rice cooked in broth until it becomes tender and creamy.

1 cup farro

1 tablespoon butter or margarine

½ cup diced white or Spanish onion

2 garlic cloves, minced

2½ cups Homemade Chicken Stock (page 61) or store-bought

1 cup chopped fresh spinach

1 cup frozen mixed peas and carrots

¼ cup whipping cream

¼ cup grated Parmesan cheese

Salt

Freshly ground black pepper

1. Place the farro in a colander and rinse in cold water.
2. In a large saucepan over medium heat, melt the butter. Add the onion and cook until the onions are translucent, about 3 minutes. Add the garlic and cook for 1 minute.
3. Raise the heat to high, add the stock and farro, and bring to a boil. Lower the heat to medium-low and simmer until all the stock is absorbed, about 15 minutes.
4. Add the spinach, frozen peas and carrots, whipping cream, and Parmesan cheese and stir to combine. Cook until heated through. Taste and season with salt and pepper. Serve hot.

Helpful Hint: If you or your family are lactose-intolerant or dairy-free, substitute almond milk, rice milk, coconut milk, soy milk, or oat milk for the whipping cream. The risotto will not be quite as creamy, but it will still be delicious. Make sure to use milk alternatives that are fortified so you get that boost of calcium.

Per serving: Calories: 330; Fat: 12g; Carbohydrates: 45g; Fiber: 7g; Protein: 14g; Sodium: 185mg; Vitamin B12: 2%; Iron: 14%

Black Bean Burgers

Serves 4

Prep time: 10 minutes / Cook time: 1 hour 15 minutes

Here is a quick and easy vegetarian burger recipe that is far healthier and better-tasting than any store-bought version. It's packed with so much flavor and fiber that you'll never miss the meat. To make this gluten-free, replace the bread crumbs and bun with gluten-free varieties. You can even wrap your burger in lettuce leaves, if you like.

FOR THE BURGER

½ cup brown rice

2 cups cold water

1 (15½-ounce) can black beans, drained and rinsed

2 green onions, finely chopped

1 garlic clove, minced

1 large egg

¼ cup bread crumbs

1 teaspoon Dijon mustard

½ teaspoon Italian seasoning

Salt

Freshly ground black pepper

4 whole-wheat burger buns

OPTIONAL TOPPINGS

Sliced onion

Sliced avocado

Sliced tomatoes

Pickle chips

Mustard

Mayonnaise

Ketchup

Relish

Lettuce of choice

1. Preheat the oven to 375°F. Line a baking sheet with parchment paper.
2. Rinse the rice in cold water until the water runs clear. Place the rice and water in a medium saucepan over high heat and bring to a boil. Lower the heat to medium-low, cover, and simmer for 50 minutes. Remove from the heat and let sit, covered, for 5 minutes. Drain any remaining water and fluff the rice with a fork.
3. In a large bowl, mash the black beans with a fork. Add the green onions, garlic, egg, bread crumbs, Dijon mustard, Italian seasoning, and rice and mix well. Season with salt and pepper.
4. Form the mixture into 4 equal patties and place them on the prepared baking sheet.
5. Bake for 20 to 25 minutes, or until heated through.

6. Serve on the buns with the optional toppings on the side.
7. Store the cooked burgers in an airtight container in the refrigerator for up to 5 days or freeze for up to 3 months.

Helpful Hint: Make a double or triple batch and freeze them, and you'll always be ready to serve dinner to lots of hungry guests.

Per serving: Calories: 220; Fat: 3g; Carbohydrates: 40g; Fiber: 8g; Protein: 10g; Sodium: 165mg; Vitamin B12: 2%; Iron: 18%

Lentil and Chicken Shepherd's Pie

Serves 6

Prep time: 15 minutes / Cook time: 1 hour

The lentils in this shepherd's pie are a great way to increase fiber in your diet. Added bonus? They also help reduce your grocery bill, as lentils are much easier on the wallet than meat.

4 russet potatoes, quartered

Salt

Freshly ground black pepper

2 tablespoons vegetable oil, divided

½ pound ground chicken, formed into a large patty

1 white or Spanish onion, finely chopped

2 garlic cloves, minced

2 cups finely chopped mushrooms

1 cup frozen mixed peas, carrots, and corn

1 (15-ounce) can lentils, drained and rinsed

1 cup Homemade Chicken Stock (page 61) or store-bought

1 tablespoon cornstarch

¼ teaspoon dried thyme

¼ teaspoon dried rosemary

1. Preheat the oven to 400°F. Grease a 9-by-13-inch baking dish.
2. In a large saucepan over high heat, place the potatoes, cover them with cold water, and bring to a boil. Lower the heat to medium and simmer until the potatoes are soft, about 15 minutes. Drain, and mash them using a potato masher or a hand mixer until smooth. Lightly season with salt and pepper and set aside.
3. In a medium saucepan over medium heat, warm 1 tablespoon of oil. Add the chicken patty and cook until it browns, about 4 minutes. Flip the patty and brown the other side, about 4 more minutes. Break up the chicken into small pieces with a spoon.
4. Add the remaining 1 tablespoon of oil and the onion, garlic, mushrooms, mixed frozen vegetables, lentils, stock, cornstarch, thyme, and rosemary and cook for 2 to 3 minutes.
5. Pour the chicken mixture into the prepared baking dish.

6. Spread the mashed potatoes evenly on top of the chicken mixture.
7. Bake for 25 to 35 minutes, or until the casserole is heated through and the potatoes begin to brown. Serve hot.
8. Store leftovers in an airtight container in the refrigerator for up to 5 days or in the freezer for up to 3 months.

Per serving: Calories: 257; Fat: 6g; Carbohydrates: 36g; Fiber: 7g; Protein: 17g; Sodium: 66mg; Vitamin B12: <1%; Iron: 17%

Meat Sauce with Lentils

Serves 6

Prep time: 10 minutes / Cook time: 30 minutes

In this sauce, the high-fiber lentils take on a similar texture and flavor to ground meat. I find it a great way to decrease your meat intake (a goal for diverticulitis sufferers) and increase your intake of some plant-based proteins. If you're looking to boost your iron, swap out the ground chicken for ground bison, which is packed with iron and is much leaner than beef. Serve this sauce over high-fiber pasta or even baked potatoes.

2 tablespoons vegetable oil, divided

½ pound ground chicken, formed into a large patty

1 white or Spanish onion, finely chopped

2 garlic cloves, minced

2 cups finely chopped mushrooms

1 tablespoon Italian seasoning

1 zucchini, grated

1 (15-ounce) can crushed tomatoes

1 (15-ounce) can lentils, drained and rinsed

Salt

Freshly ground black pepper

1. In a large saucepan over medium heat, warm 1 tablespoon of oil. Add the chicken patty and cook until it browns, about 4 minutes. Flip the patty and brown the other side, another 4 minutes. Break up the chicken into small pieces with a spoon.
2. Add the remaining 1 tablespoon of oil and the onion, garlic, mushrooms, and Italian seasoning and cook for 2 to 3 minutes.
3. Add the zucchini, tomatoes, and lentils and simmer, stirring frequently, for 15 to 20 minutes. Taste and season with salt and pepper. Serve hot.
4. Store leftovers in airtight containers in the refrigerator for up to 5 days or in the freezer for up to 3 months.

Per serving: Calories: 198; Fat: 8g; Carbohydrates: 18g; Fiber: 7g; Protein: 16g; Sodium: 139mg; Vitamin B12: <1%; Iron: 16%

Guacamole

Serves 6

Prep time: 10 minutes

Nothing makes me think of warm summer days like fresh guacamole. Not only are avocados delicious, they are also packed with fiber and heart-healthy fats. Spread this guac onto sandwiches, toast, or whole-grain tortillas.

4 avocados
¼ cup diced red onion
2 plum tomatoes, diced
¼ cup chopped fresh cilantro
2 tablespoons fresh lime juice
Pinch ground cumin
Hot sauce
Salt
Freshly ground black pepper

1. In a medium bowl, mash the avocados with a fork.
2. Gently stir in the red onion, tomatoes, cilantro, lime juice, cumin, and a splash of hot sauce. Taste and season with salt, pepper, and additional hot sauce, if desired.
3. Serve with high-fiber tortilla chips, cut-up vegetables, or high-fiber crackers.

Per serving (guacamole only): Calories: 202; Fat: 18g; Carbohydrates: 12g; Fiber: 8g; Protein: 3g; Sodium: 13mg; Vitamin B12: 0%; Iron: 5%

Homemade Hummus

Serves 4

Prep time: 10 minutes

Hummus is a popular dish in the Middle East and Mediterranean countries. This creamy dish is packed with dietary fiber and can be found in grocery stores everywhere, but it is so easy to make and tastes so good. Plus, there won't be any chemicals or preservatives. Chickpeas (also called garbanzo beans) are a rich source of fiber, folate, iron, phosphorus, and zinc.

1 (15-ounce) can chickpeas

2 garlic cloves, roughly chopped

4 tablespoons tahini

2 tablespoons extra-virgin olive oil

1 tablespoon lemon juice

½ teaspoon ground cumin

2 tablespoons water

Salt

Freshly ground black pepper

1. Place the chickpeas, garlic, tahini, olive oil, lemon juice, cumin, and water in a blender or food processor and puree until smooth. Taste and season with salt and pepper.
2. Serve with cut-up vegetables, high-fiber crackers, or whole-wheat pita on the side.

Per serving (hummus only) ¼ cup: Calories: 278; Fat: 16g; Carbohydrates: 28g; Fiber: 6g; Protein: 8g; Sodium: 333mg; Vitamin B12: 0%; Iron: 17%

Bean Salad

Serves 4

Prep time: 10 minutes

Try this salad for a change of pace from potato salad at the next family barbecue, summer picnic, or potluck. It's colorful, loaded with fiber, and really tasty.

FOR THE DRESSING

¼ cup vegetable oil

2 tablespoons lime juice

1 tablespoon chopped fresh cilantro

1 teaspoon honey

½ teaspoon Dijon mustard

1 garlic clove, minced

Salt

Freshly ground black pepper

FOR THE SALAD

1 (15½-ounce) can chickpeas, drained and rinsed

1 (15½-ounce) can black beans, drained and rinsed

1 (15-ounce) can kidney beans, drained and rinsed

1 cup diced cucumber

¾ cup canned corn

2 tablespoons diced red onion

½ avocado, diced

To make the dressing

1. In a small bowl, whisk together the oil, lime juice, cilantro, honey, Dijon mustard, and garlic. Taste and season with salt and pepper.

To make the salad

2. In a medium bowl, mix together the chickpeas, black beans, kidney beans, cucumber, corn, red onion, and avocado. Add the dressing and lightly toss. Serve immediately.
3. Store the salad in an airtight container in the refrigerator for up to 5 days.

Per serving: Calories: 518; Fat: 20g; Carbohydrates: 72g; Fiber: 21g; Protein: 19g; Sodium: 559mg; Vitamin B12: 0%; Iron: 33%

Greek Farro Salad

Serves 6

Prep time: 10 minutes / Cook time: 25 minutes

If you love Greek salad, try this twist: I've taken a classic Greek salad and added farro, creating a high-fiber meal that tastes as good as it looks.

FOR THE DRESSING

¼ cup olive oil

1 tablespoon red wine vinegar

¼ teaspoon dried oregano

¼ teaspoon garlic powder

½ teaspoon Dijon mustard

Salt

Freshly ground black pepper

FOR THE SALAD

1½ cups farro

5 cups cold water

1 cup diced English cucumber

¼ cup diced red onion

1 red bell pepper, diced

1 (15½-ounce) can chickpeas, drained and rinsed

½ cup halved cherry tomatoes

½ cup Kalamata olives

½ cup crumbled feta cheese

To make the dressing

1. In a small bowl, whisk together the oil, vinegar, oregano, garlic powder, and Dijon mustard. Taste and season with salt and pepper.

To make the salad

2. In a large saucepan over high heat, mix together the farro and water and bring to a boil. Lower the heat to medium-low and cook until tender, 15 to 20 minutes. Set aside and let cool.

3. In a medium bowl, mix together the farro, cucumber, red onion, bell pepper, chickpeas, tomatoes, olives, and feta. Pour in the dressing and lightly toss. Serve immediately.

Per serving: Calories: 371; Fat: 14g; Carbohydrates: 52g; Fiber: 11g; Protein: 13g; Sodium: 307mg; Vitamin B12: 4%; Iron: 20%

Baked Pears with Homemade Granola

Serves 8

Prep time: 10 minutes / Cook time: 40 minutes

Enjoy this nice light treat when you're craving something sweet. This recipe looks fancy, but it takes very little time to make. It's perfect for dinner parties or date night (just cut the recipe in half; you'll still have leftovers!).

FOR THE GRANOLA

1 cup rolled oats

¼ cup almonds

1 tablespoon chia seeds

1 tablespoon hemp seeds

1 tablespoon pumpkin or sunflower seeds

½ teaspoon ground cinnamon

Pinch salt

1 tablespoon coconut oil, melted

2 teaspoons maple syrup

¼ teaspoon vanilla extract

FOR THE PEARS

4 Anjou pears

½ cup maple syrup

1 teaspoon vanilla extract

½ teaspoon ground cinnamon

To make the granola

1. Preheat the oven to 375°F. Line a baking sheet with parchment paper.
2. In a large bowl, mix together the oats, almonds, chia seeds, hemp seeds, pumpkin seeds, cinnamon, and salt.
3. In a small bowl, mix together the coconut oil, maple syrup, and vanilla. Drizzle the mixture over the oat mixture and stir to combine.
4. Spread the oat mixture out onto the prepared baking sheet. Bake for 10 minutes and stir well. Continue to bake for another 10 minutes. Let cool on a wire rack.

continued ▸

Baked Pears with Homemade Granola continued

To make the pears

5. Line the baking sheet with another sheet of parchment paper.
6. Cut the pears in half lengthwise. Cut a very small slice off the rounded side of each half, which will help the pears sit flat. Using a melon baller or a spoon, scoop out the core and seeds. Place the pear halves on the prepared baking sheet.
7. Spoon the granola into the pears.
8. In a small bowl, whisk together the maple syrup and vanilla and drizzle it over the pears. Sprinkle the cinnamon over the pear halves.
9. Bake for 15 to 20 minutes, or until the pears are cooked through and tender. Serve immediately.

Per serving: Calories: 196; Fat: 2g; Carbohydrates: 34g; Fiber: 5g; Protein: 4g; Sodium: 5mg; Vitamin B12: 0%; Iron: 9%

Avocado Chia Pudding Four Ways

Serves 4

Prep time: 10 minutes / Set time: 2 hours

You had me at pudding! This is a healthier version of pudding with avocado for added creaminess and fiber-rich chia, which gives it a pudding-like texture. Make the base recipe and choose one of the four variations to flavor it however you like.

FOR THE PUDDING BASE

2 cups milk of choice

½ avocado, mashed

½ cup chia seeds

3 tablespoons honey, plus more as needed

½ teaspoon vanilla extract

FLAVOR OPTIONS

CHOCOLATE

¼ cup unsweetened cocoa powder

PUMPKIN SPICE

½ cup pumpkin puree

1 teaspoon ground cinnamon

¼ teaspoon ground ginger

Pinch ground cloves

APPLE PIE

½ cup applesauce

1 teaspoon ground cinnamon

¼ teaspoon ground ginger

Pinch ground cloves

BERRY

½ cup berries of choice

1. Put the milk, avocado, chia seeds, honey, and vanilla in a food processor or a blender and puree until smooth. Taste, and add more honey, if desired.
2. Add the ingredients for your choice of flavors and puree.
3. Pour the mixture into bowls or mason jars, cover, and refrigerate for at least 2 hours.

Per serving for the base: Calories: 257; Fat: 11g; Carbohydrates: 31g; Fiber: 12g; Protein: 11g; Sodium: 56mg; Vitamin B12: 9%; Iron: 13%

Dark Chocolate Brownies

Makes 9 brownies

Prep time: 10 minutes / Cook time: 35 minutes

Dark chocolate is naturally high in iron, but it becomes even more nutritious when paired with black beans. You might be making these for the health benefits, but everyone will love them for how rich and decadent they are.

- **¾ cup dark chocolate chips**
- **8 tablespoons (1 stick) butter or margarine**
- **½ (15½-ounce) can black beans, drained and rinsed**
- **½ cup sugar**
- **2 large eggs**
- **2 teaspoons vanilla extract**
- **1¾ cups whole-wheat flour**
- **2 tablespoons unsweetened dark cocoa powder**
- **Pinch salt**

1. Preheat the oven to 350°F. Line a 9-by-9-inch square baking pan with aluminum foil or parchment paper and grease well. Set aside.
2. In a microwave-safe bowl, melt the chocolate chips and butter in the microwave in 20-second intervals, stirring occasionally, until smooth. Let cool.
3. In a blender, puree the beans, adding water 1 teaspoon at a time, until smooth. Set aside.
4. Add the sugar to the cooled chocolate and whisk to combine. Whisk in the eggs, one at a time. Add the vanilla and pureed black beans and stir to combine.
5. Gradually mix in the flour, cocoa powder, and salt until well combined.
6. Pour the batter into the prepared pan, spreading it evenly. Bake for 30 to 35 minutes, or until a toothpick inserted into the middle comes clean. Let cool completely in the pan on a wire rack. Remove the brownies from the pan by lifting the foil. Cut into 9 bars.

7. Let stand at room temperature for at least 30 minutes before serving.
8. Store the brownies wrapped in plastic wrap at room temperature for up to 2 days or in the refrigerator for up to 4 months.

Per serving (1 brownie): Calories: 301; Fat: 13g; Carbohydrates: 42g; Fiber: 6g; Protein: 6g; Sodium: 106mg; Vitamin B12: 2%; Iron: 12%

Chocolate Chip Protein Bites

Makes 10 protein bites
Prep time: 10 minutes

When you have a craving for dessert, eat one of these. The protein, fiber, and fat from the nut butter, chia, hemp, and flax help keep you feeling full, and they are sweet enough to curb that longing for sugar.

½ cup Rice Krispies
½ cup natural nut butter
½ cup rolled oats
⅓ cup ground flaxseed
¼ cup honey or maple syrup
2 tablespoons hemp seeds
1 tablespoon chia seeds
1 tablespoon chocolate chips
1 teaspoon vanilla extract
½ teaspoon ground cinnamon

1. In a large bowl, mix together the Rice Krispies, nut butter, oats, flaxseed, honey, hemp seeds, chia seeds, chocolate chips, vanilla, and cinnamon until well combined.
2. Using your hands, roll the mixture into 10 balls. If the mixture is really sticky, wear food-safe plastic gloves to roll them.
3. Store the balls in an airtight container in the freezer for up to 3 months.

Per serving (1 protein bite): Calories: 166; Fat: 10g; Carbohydrates: 16g; Fiber: 3g; Protein: 5g; Sodium: 70mg; Vitamin B12: 3%; Iron: 7%

Oat Bars with Raspberry Chia Jam

Makes 9 bars

Prep time: 15 minutes / Cook time: 25 minutes

Soft and chewy, these healthy oat bars have a wonderful raspberry jam filling made with chia seeds, our high-fiber friend.

FOR THE JAM

1 cup frozen raspberries

2 tablespoons chia seeds

1 tablespoon honey

1 teaspoon vanilla extract

FOR THE OAT BARS

2 cups whole-wheat flour

1⅓ cups rolled oats

1 cup brown sugar

1 cup (2 sticks) butter or margarine, at room temperature

2 teaspoons ground cinnamon

1 teaspoon vanilla extract

To make the jam

1. In a microwave-safe bowl, heat the raspberries in the microwave, in 1-minute intervals, until soft.
2. Add the chia seeds, honey, and vanilla and let sit until thickened, about 5 minutes.

To make the oat bars

3. Preheat the oven to 350°F. Grease an 8-by-8-inch baking dish. Set aside.
4. In a large bowl, mix together the flour, oats, brown sugar, butter, cinnamon, and vanilla.
5. Press about two-thirds of the mixture into the prepared baking dish. Using a spoon, spread the chia jam over the oat mixture, leaving a ½-inch space around the edges to prevent the jam from burning when it's baked.

continued ▸

Oat Bars with Raspberry Chia Jam continued

6. Sprinkle the remaining oat mixture over the jam.
7. Bake for 20 to 25 minutes, or until the bars are golden brown. Let cool completely on a wire rack.
8. Once cooled, cut into 9 bars and serve.

Helpful Hint: These taste really great topped with a scoop of vanilla ice cream. Or serve them for breakfast with a spoonful of plain or vanilla Greek yogurt.

Per serving (1 bar): Calories: 407; Fat: 22g; Carbohydrates: 51g; Fiber: 6g; Protein: 6g; Sodium: 152mg; Vitamin B12: 1%; Iron: 14%

Resources

American Society of Colon and Rectal Surgeons
(fascrs.org/patients/diseases-and-conditions/a-z/diverticular-disease)

Canadian Digestive Health Foundation
(cdhf.ca/digestive-disorders/diverticular-disease)

Canadian Society of Intestinal Research
(badgut.org/information-centre/a-z-digestive-topics
/diverticular-disease)

National Institute of Diabetes and Digestive and Kidney Diseases
(niddk.nih.gov/health-information/digestive-diseases
/diverticulosis-diverticulitis)

References

Academy of Nutrition and Dietetics. "Fibre Content of Foods." *Nutrition Care Manual*. nutritioncaremanual.org.

Aldoori, Walid, and Milly Ryan-Harshman. "Preventing Diverticular Disease: Review of Recent Evidence on High-Fibre Diets." *Canadian Family Physician* 48, no. 10 (October 2002): 1632–37. cfp.ca/content/48/10/1632.

American College of Gastroenterology. "Diverticulosis and Diverticulitis." Accessed January 22, 2016. gi.org/topics/diverticulosis-and-diverticulitis.

Arasaradnam, R. P., D. Commane, H. Greetham, M. Bradburn, I. T. Johnson, and J. C. Mathers. "A Novel Finding—Global DNA Hypomethylation in Diverticular Disease: A Pilot Study (the BORICC Study)." *Gut* 56, supplement no. 2 (April 2007): A44–45. gut.bmj.com/content/56/suppl_2.

Bogardus, Sidney T., Jr. "What Do We Know about Diverticular Disease? A Brief Overview." *Journal of Clinical Gastroenterology* 40, supplement no. 3 (August 2006): S108–11. doi:10.1097/01.mcg.0000212603.28595.5c.

"Diverticulitis." University of California San Francisco Center for Colorectal Surgery. May 2016.

Dobbins, C., D. DeFontgalland, G. Duthie, and D. A. Wattchow. "The Relationship of Obesity to the Complications of Diverticular Disease." *Colorectal Disease* 8, no. 1 (January 2006): 37-40. doi:10.1111/j.1463-1318.2005.00847.x.

Dughera, L., A. M. Serra, E. Battaglia, D. Tibaudi, M. Navino, and G. Emanuelli. "Acute Recurrent Diverticulitis Is Prevented by Oral Administration of a Polybacterial Lysate Suspension." *Minerva gastroenterologica e dietologica* 50, no. 2 (June 2004): 149–54. minervamedica.it/en/journals/gastroenterologica-dietologica/article.php?cod=R08Y2004N02A0149.

Floch, Martin H., and Jonathan A. White. "Management of Diverticular Disease Is Changing." *World Journal of Gastroenterology* 12, no. 20 (May 28, 2006): 3225–28. doi:10.3748/wjg.v12.i20.3225.

Goh, H., and R. Bourne. "Non-steroidal Anti-inflammatory Drugs and Perforated Diverticular Disease: A Case-Control Study." *Annals of the Royal College of Surgeons of England* 84, no. 2 (March 2002): 93–96. ncbi.nlm.nih.gov/pmc/articles/PMC2503782.

Grahn, Sarah W., and Madhulika G. Varma. "Factors That Increase Risk of Colon Polyps." *Clinics in Colon and Rectal Surgery* 21, no. 4 (November 2008): 247–55. doi:10.1055/s-0028-1089939.

Harvard Health Publishing. "Diverticular Disease of the Colon." Last modified December 20, 2018. health.harvard.edu /diseases-and-conditions/diverticular-disease-of-the-colon.

Lakatos, P. L. "Environmental Factors Affecting Inflammatory Bowel Disease: Have We Made Progress?" *Digestive Diseases* 27, no. 3 (September 2009): 215–25. doi:10/1159/000228553.

Makola, Diklar. "Diverticular Disease: Evidence for Dietary Intervention?" Nutrition Issues in Gastroenterology Series, no. 47. *Practical Gastroenterology* (February 2007): 38–46. med.virginia.edu /ginutrition/wp-content/uploads/sites/199/2015/11/Makola Article-Feb-07.pdf.

Onur, Mehmet Ruhi, Erhan Akpinar, Ali Devrum Karaosmanoglu, Cavid Isayev, and Musturay Karcaaltincaba. "Diverticulitis: A Comprehensive Review with Usual and Unusual Complications." *Insights into Imaging* 8, no. 1 (February 2017): 19–27. doi:10.1007 /s13244-016-0532-3.

Painter, Neil S., and Denis P. Burkitt. "Diverticular Disease of the Colon: A Deficiency Disease of Western Civilization." *British Medical Journal* 2, no. 5759 (May 22, 1971): 450–54. doi:10.1136/bmj.2.5759.450.

Peery, Anne F., Tope O. Keku, Christopher F. Martin, Swathi Eluri, Thomas Runge, Joseph A. Galanko, and Robert S. Sandler. "Distribution and Characteristics of Colonic Diverticula in a United States Screening Population." *Clinical Gastroenterology and Hepatology* 14, no. 7 (July 2016): 980–85.e1. doi:10.1016/j.cgh.2016.01.020.

Reichert, Matthias C., and Frank Lammert. "The Genetic Epidemiology of Diverticulosis and Diverticular Disease: Emerging Evidence." *United European Gastroenterology Journal* 3, no. 5 (October 2015): 409–18. doi:10.1177/2050640615576676.

Shahedi, Kamyar, Garth Fuller, Roger Bolus, Erica Cohen, Michelle Vu, Rena Shah, Nikhil Agarwal, et al. "Long-Term Risk of Acute Diverticulitis among Patients with Incidental Diverticulosis Found during Colonoscopy." *Clinical Gastroenterology and Hepatology* 11, no. 12 (December 2013): 1609–13. doi:10.1016/j.cgh.2013.06.020.

Strate, Lisa L., Yan L. Liu, Edward S. Huang, Edward L. Giovannucci, and Andrew T. Chan. "Use of Aspirin or Nonsteroidal Anti-inflammatory Drugs Increases Risk for Diverticulitis and Diverticular Bleeding." *Gastroenterology* 140, no. 5 (May 2011): 1427–33. doi:10.1053/j.gastro.2011.02.004.

Strate, Lisa L., Yan L. Liu, Walid H. Aldoori, and Edward L. Giovannucci. "Physical Activity Decreases Diverticular Complications." *American Journal of Gastroenterology* 104, no. 5 (May 2009): 1221–30. doi:10.1038/ajg.2009.121.

Tarleton, Sherry, and John K. DiBaise. "Low-Residue Diet in Diverticular Disease: Putting an End to a Myth." *Nutrition in Clinical Practice* 26, no. 2 (April 2011): 137–42. doi:10.1177/0884533611399774.

Tolstrup, Janne Schurmann, Louise Kristiansen, and Ulrik Becker. "Smoking and Risk of Acute and Chronic Pancreatitis among Women and Men: A Population-Based Cohort Study." *Archives of Internal Medicine* 169, no. 6 (March 23, 2009): 603–9. doi:10.1001/archinternmed.2008.601.

Tursi, Antonio. "Efficacy, Safety, and Applicability of Outpatient Treatment for Diverticulitis." *Drug, Healthcare and Patient Safety* 6 (2014): 29–36. doi:10.2147/DHPS.S61277.

Tursi, Antonio, Giovanni Brandimarte, Gian Marco Giorgetti, and Walter Elisei. "Mesalazine and/or *Lactobacillus casei* in Preventing Recurrence of Symptomatic Uncomplicated Diverticular Disease of the Colon: A Prospective, Randomized, Open-Label Study." *Journal of Clinical Gastroenterology* 40, no. 4 (April 2006): 312–16. doi:10.1097/01.mcg.0000210092.77296.6d.

Weizman, Adam V., and Geoffrey C. Nguyen. "Diverticular Disease: Epidemiology and Management." *Canadian Journal of Gastroenterology and Hepatology* 25, no. 7 (July 2011): 385–89. doi:10.1155/2011/795241.

Wheat, Chelle L., and Lisa L. Strate. "Trends in Hospitalization for Diverticulitis and Diverticular Bleeding in the United States from 2000 to 2010." *Clinical Gastroenterology and Hepatology* 14, no. 1 (January 2016): 96–103.e1. doi:10.1016/j.cgh.2015.03.030.

Williams, Paul T. "Incident Diverticular Disease Is Inversely Related to Vigorous Physical Activity." *Medicine and Science in Sports and Exercise* 41, no. 5 (May 2009): 1042–47. doi:10.1249/MSS.0b013e318192d02d.

Index

C

D

E

N

O

P

Q

R

S

T

V

W

Y

Z

Acknowledgments

I'm very grateful and fortunate to have an amazing community of supportive dietitians always in my corner. Thank you to my wonderful coworkers, friends, and family for the encouragement and support throughout this amazing journey.

A special thank-you to my mentors, Chef Margaret Turner and Mary-Sue Waisman, RD. I am forever grateful for your words of encouragement and guidance in the early stages of my career and support as I transitioned from the culinary world to the world of nutrition. I cannot thank you enough for helping me find the most amazing and rewarding career, which I love.

Finally, thank you to Callisto Media editor Reina Glenn for recognizing the need for a book to help provide support to those diagnosed with diverticulitis.

About the Author

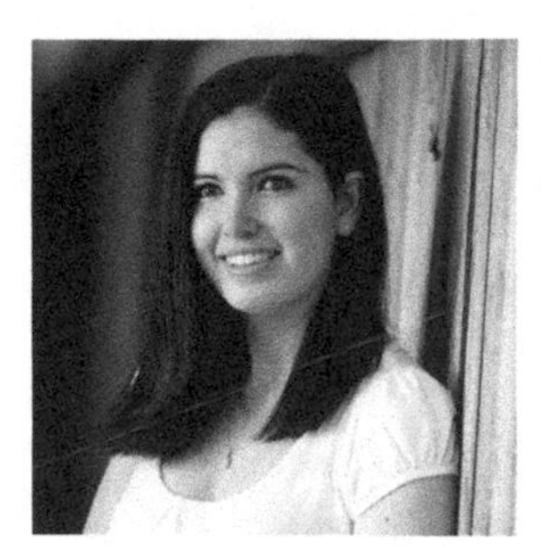

Karyn Sunohara, RD, is a chef, speaker, and writer who specializes in digestive health, pediatrics, cancer, eating disorders, and culinary nutrition. Karyn loves to give her clients practical nutrition tips and recipes to help them reach their health and nutrition goals.

Karyn has provided nutrition counseling, cooking classes, and education to thousands of people between the work she does at South Calgary Primary Care Network, Wellspring Calgary, Ignite Nutrition, and her private practice For the LOVE of FOOD, in Calgary, Canada. You can follow her new recipe creations on her Instagram account at for_the_love_of_f00d or on her website at forthel0veoffood.weebly.com.

When Karyn's not working with her clients, you can find her in the kitchen writing new recipes, spending time with her nieces and nephews, fishing with her partner Rob, or spending time with her fur children.